Birth in
ANCIENT CHINA

SUNY series in Chinese Philosophy and Culture
———————
Roger T. Ames, editor

Birth in ANCIENT CHINA

A Study of Metaphor and Cultural Identity
in Pre-Imperial China

Constance A. Cook and Xinhui Luo

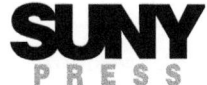

Cover image of face from Hongshun ritual site. Photo by Tian Shuai. Courtesy of the National Museum of China.

Published by State University of New York Press, Albany

© 2017 State University of New York

All rights reserved

Printed in the United States of America

No part of this book may be used or reproduced in any manner whatsoever without written permission. No part of this book may be stored in a retrieval system or transmitted in any form or by any means including electronic, electrostatic, magnetic tape, mechanical, photocopying, recording, or otherwise without the prior permission in writing of the publisher.

For information, contact State University of New York Press, Albany, NY
www.sunypress.edu

Production, Ryan Morris
Marketing, Kate R. Seburyamo

Library of Congress Cataloging-in-Publication Data

Names: Cook, Constance A., author. | Luo, Xinhui, co-author.
Title: Birth in ancient China : a study of metaphor and cultural identity in pre-imperial China / Constance A. Cook and Luo Xinhui.
Description: Albany : State University of New York Press, [2017] | Series: SUNY series in Chinese philosophy and culture | Includes bibliographical references and index.
Identifiers: LCCN 2016054534 (print) | LCCN 2016057612 (ebook) | ISBN 9781438467115 (hardcover : alkaline paper) | ISBN 9781438467108 (pbk : alk. paper) | ISBN 9781438467122 (ebook)
Subjects: LCSH: Childbirth—Social aspects—China—History—To 1500. | Birth customs—China—History—To 1500. | Human reproduction—Social aspects—China—History—To 1500. | Metaphor—Social aspects—China—History—To 1500. | Group identity—China—History—To 1500. | China—Social life and customs—To 221 B.C. | China—History—Zhou dynasty, 1122–221 B.C.
Classification: LCC GN482.1 .C66 2017 (print) | LCC GN482.1 (ebook) | DDC 392.1/2—dc23
LC record available at https://lccn.loc.gov/2016054534

10 9 8 7 6 5 4 3 2 1

Contents

List of Illustrations	vii
Acknowledgments	ix
Introduction: A Chu Text	xi
Chapter 1. Words and Images	1
Chu Ancestral Names and the Word for Birth	5
A Lost Word for Birth	9
Suggestive Images	11
Chapter 2. Controlling Reproduction: Fertility Prayers	21
Zhou Fertility Prayers in Bronze Inscriptions	23
A Warring States Prayer Preserved on Bamboo Strips	29
Chapter 3. Mothers and Embryos	43
Embryonic Transformation	47
Chapter 4. Controlling the Pregnant Body	53
Time and Divination	53
Curses, Stars, and the Gendered Cosmos	63
Sequestering	68
A Question of Thorns	73
Chapter 5. Divine Origins and Chu Genealogical History	75
Gender-Bending	89
Chapter 6. The Traumatic Births of Non-Zhou Ancestral Founders	93

Conclusion	109
Notes	111
Bibliography	131
Index	149

Illustrations

Chart 1.	Shang and later graphs for embodiment	3
Chart 2.	Shang words related to birthing	4
Chart 3.	Chu progenitor names and related graphs	6
Figure 1.	Hongshan sculpture of a pregnant body	11
Figure 2.	Banpo pottery bowl paintings with baby faces	12
Figure 3.	Possible fertility symbolism on a Neolithic pot	13
Figure 4.	Fu Hao jade amulets with possible fertility symbolism	14
Figure 5.	Jade figurine of a woman in the birthing position	14
Figure 6.	Jade figurine of a woman with tattoos and a bird tail from Fu Hao's tomb	15
Figure 7.	Humans in the mouths of tigers, images from bronzes	16
Figure 8.	Jade amulet with a fetal-like birdman from the Fu Hao tomb site	17
Figure 9.	Figures with split bodies found on the inner coffin of Zeng Hou Yi	18
Figure 10.	Fuxi and Nüwa with snake tails and holding the sun and moon	19
Figure 11.	Oracle bones with birth divination from *Heji* 14001 and 14002	54
Chart 4.	Sequestering images	71
Chart 5.	Chu ancestral names	91
Chart 6.	Images of technical intervention in pregnancy	95

Acknowledgments

Constance Cook is grateful for the support of the International Consortium for Research in the Humanities, Friedrich-Alexander-Universität Erlangen-Nürnberg, Germany. Both authors wish to thank Tian Shuai and Hu Wenjia for their research help.

Introduction
A Chu Text

Birth is naturally a gendered phenomenon. Only a "mother" can give birth and only people labeled "females" can be mothers. In this sense, the idea of womanhood has always been intimately associated with the physical reproduction of society. Reproduction of society, history, and the ability to have a future all relied on women.[1] However, the categorization of birth as a female experience was not absolute in ancient China. For example, in Chinese philosophical and historical discourse, the vocabulary for "birth" could be used in a genderless and abstract sense of one cosmic process generating another or even a male dynastic founder producing heirs. In this book, we focus on the female experience of physical birth but, since we are necessarily limited to written texts, we also interrogate the seeming genderless aspects of mythical, philosophical, and religious contexts. Unlike other studies of female reproduction and the control over reproduction during the imperial, particularly the late-imperial, times, a study of childbirth in pre-imperial China must tease information out of ancient vocabulary and cryptic texts.[2] The heavy hand of later editors, particularly those of Han and later Ru or Confucian scholars, upon pre-imperial texts requires us to balance information provided by recently discovered bamboo and silk texts and other excavated texts, such as bone and bronze inscribed texts, against what is preserved in the transmitted classics. Material culture—that is, artifacts and burial data—can also provide hints.

The text, the *Chu ju*, that inspired this analysis of the female birth process is a recently discovered fourth-century BCE bamboo manuscript that likely originated from the middle Yangzi region, a product of a Chu 楚 scribe (the text is translated at the end of the introduction and analyzed in more detail in chapter 5). Its exact origin is unknown since it is among the historic, poetic, and divinatory texts preserved by Tsinghua University that were originally stolen by thieves from an ancient tomb. This text clearly connects birthing to lineage creation and political identity. It is remarkable because it not only provides a history of the mostly male Chu royal lineage in rhythmical prose and all its capitals up to 381 BCE, but it also includes the earliest detailed description of a female traumatic birthing experience, one that in modern times would be understood as a cesarean section. We explore the connection between birthing myths and royal genealogy as well as the cultural symbolism of the cutting or splitting open of the mother's body. But first, to put this Chu text into a larger religious and mythical context, we examine the earliest records, those produced by the Shang people during the second millennium BCE up through the time of the third-century BCE Chu text. The elite wished to control fertility, the success of the pregnancy, as well as the gender and future prognosis of the baby. Because of the religious belief structure at the time, this process included appeals to the supernatural. China's earliest birthing records are mostly preserved in divination records, oracle bones, and bamboo stalk divination manuals and almanacs, or *Day Books* (*Rishu* 日書), as well as in silk medical manuscripts and some transmitted texts.

In chapter 1, we begin our discussion with the earliest vocabulary and images associated with birth. We show the connection between the idea of human embodiment and early notions of "enclosure." In chapter 2, we discuss the efforts to control social reproduction through divination, prayers, and sacrifices to the ancestors. We also touch on the issue of birthplace and hints regarding the need to sequester the birth event, which in later times we know was to control spiritual pollution from fluids and blood. In chapter 3, we examine the idea of the "mother" as a channel of cosmic reproduction and transformation and look at ancient notions of embryonic development. In chapter 4, we examine ancient divination and other methods used to determine the outcome of birth. In chapter 5, we compare transmitted versions of Chu genealogy with that recorded in the fourth-century BCE *Chu ju* 楚居 account and pay particular attention to the role of mothers and goddesses. In chapter 6, we compare the legends of good and bad births and their cultural affiliations and note how cultural conflicts ironically preserve evidence for early surgical procedures for difficult births. Through a subtle examination of early Chinese materials, our overall study teases out the unknown history of ancient womanhood and women's role in the social reproduction of early Chinese patriarchy.

Although the ideas in this book are necessarily speculative, we feel that the Chu text provides us a unique opportunity to explore an untouched and for many a still untouchable topic: the female experience of childbirth. In the *Chu ju* text, which we will explain in detail in chapter 5, we find a number of avenues for exploration: divine genealogies, the mention of birth mothers, the contrast between a smooth versus difficult birthing, the significance of twins, the manipulations of the traumatic birth by a shaman-physician, the idea of the mother's body "splitting," and the naming of a people (the Chu people) from a tool used in the birthing of the ancestral progenitor of the Chu people and to represent their identity.[3] We analyze the meaning behind the names of these ancestors in terms of the larger birthing narrative in early China.

Only the first section of the *Chu ju* mentions the role of birth mothers in the creation of a people. The rest of the manuscript is presumably devoted to male rulers and the names of their capitals. We are concerned with the initial section. Although scholars still debate how to read some of the archaic graphs, since the content of this text frames all the discussions in this book, we first provide an English translation and follow this with a detailed analysis with the Chinese in chapter 5:

> Ji Lian at first descended onto Gui Mountain going to Xueqiong (a cave). Once he came out (from Xueqiong) to Qiao Mountain, he resided at Huanpo (a slope). Then he went up the Chuan River and had an audience with Pan Geng's daughter, who resided at Fang Mountain. Her name was Ancestress Wei ("Bird"?) and she had grasped the virtue of compassion. She wandered throughout the Four Regions. Ji Lian heard that she sought marriage, so he pursued her as far as Pan. Thereupon, she gave birth to Ying Bo (Elder Son Ying) and Yuan Zhong (Middle Son Yuan). The delivery was normal and auspicious. From early on they resided in Jingzong (Capital-Main Shrine).
>
> Later on, Xue Yin (Ji Lian's descendant, a third son, "Cave Drinker") journeyed to Jingzong, whereupon he heard about Ancestress Lie ("Break Apart," or Li) in the Zai River region. She was mature with long delicate ears, so he took her as a wife and she gave birth to Dou Shu (Middle Sibling Dou) and Li Ji (Youngest Son Li). Li did not follow (Shu down the birth canal) but came out through a split in her side. Ancestress Lie's (spirit) went to visit Heaven. Shaman

Xian cut into (sewed? wrapped? confronted the demon in?) her side with a thorn(s?), hence the modern term *chu ren* 楚人, "the People of the Thorns."

The complex imagery of meeting the young women in wild areas of mountains and rivers, of their smooth versus traumatic birthing of twins, of the use of thorns by shamans, and even the names of the people and places mentioned will be explored in greater detail in the following chapters. First, however, we will set up the social and religious context in which this tale of the birth of a people was imagined.

1

Words and Images

For the root sense of childbirth, we will look at the first written words and the earliest images. The first written words appear on Shang oracle bones dated at the earliest to the thirteenth century BCE, about the time of suggestive decor on bronze sacrificial vessels. Both text and imagery were tied to the Shang ancestor worship system and thus were fundamental to what evolved into a sophisticated Central Plains civilization, which had spread by the beginning of imperial times in the late third century BCE throughout the middle and lower valleys of the Yellow and Yangzi Rivers. The earliest images suggestive of a concern for childbirth and fertility and, hence, social reproduction date back to the early Neolithic period, around the fifth millennium BCE. Although these prehistoric cultures may have had an influence on what became Shang civilization, the eras are too distant to make direct cultural links. However, we include some of these, since they appeared within the borders of modern China and may have contributed in some fashion to later culture layers. Although these artifacts occurred at sites geographically peripheral to where the Shang would rise in power (the modern city of Anyang in Henan Province), they represent colorful aspects of the East Asian heartland's past. On the other hand, even the Shang bronze decor from Anyang seems somewhat alien from the texts, especially the later texts, and thus remains only suggestive of larger conceptual frameworks.

A number of graphs represent the human and human body in ancient texts (see chart 1 for reference). One graph seems to depict a side view of a person bent over with arms outstretched, an image that can be read as a living "human" or "person" (ren 人) or as a group of people associated with a place or lineage.¹ The archaic graph for "person" is slightly different from the graph with the bend in the opposite direction, which is read as "dead person" or "corpse" (shi 尸). The next two graphs in the chart represent female and male ancestors. The former (bi 匕 for 妣) is an image of a "person" holding some sort of implement. The latter (且 for zu 祖) is a phallic image. Graphs related to "person" in the next two lines include "body" (shen 身) and "pregnancy" (yun 孕). The earliest recorded texts, on Shang oracle bones, talk about the body mostly in terms of supernaturally afflicted illness. Was it a curse from a particular ancestral spirit, such as Father Yi 乙 or Ancestress Ji 己? Should they present an exorcism sacrifice to Ancestor Ding? A graph depicting the body with a baby represented the verb and condition of "becoming or being pregnant." An affair of great concern to the Shang king and his diviners was whether a particular wife would become pregnant and whether the pregnancy would successfully produce a male heir. Variations of the graphic representation of pregnancy include ones emphasizing the female aspect of the body with folded arms or a belly, standing or seated. These variations are seen as enhancements of the graphs for female and mother (see the next line in chart 1). "Mother" 母 was sometimes distinguished from "woman" 女 by marks indicating her breasts. Generally, the graph for "woman" (without the breast marks) was used in names or to mark the gender of a baby. The term "mother" as marked with the breasts was generally applied to recently deceased elite women, who as mothers of lineage heirs could receive sacrifice from their descendants.²

In later times, the graphs for body and pregnancy became somewhat confused. In the late Western Zhou period (late ninth through mid-eighth century BCE), for example, variants of the graph for "body" (shen) might include just a dot in the protruding belly (see the bronze inscription examples in chart 1). By this time, too, the graph represented the word for one's "person" or "self," and it becomes increasingly abstract over time.³ Interestingly, the ancient pronunciations of the words for pregnancy (*liŋ-s), body (*ɲiŋ), and human being (*niŋ) were quite close, suggesting perhaps that pregnancy was seen as a cognate extension of the embodiment of self.⁴

There were two ancient graphs that meant "to give birth" (see chart 2 on page 4). One used commonly in later times (yu 毓) was used rarely in Shang times in the direct sense of a female giving birth (top line in chart 2). But because of its relationship to ancestors' names and genealogy, we discuss it first. The Shang word more often used for "to

Chart 1. Shang and later graphs for embodiment

Person (人 *niŋ)

Corpse (尸 *lˤ[ə]j)

Female ancestor (妣 *pijʔ)

Male ancestor (祖 *[ts]ˤaʔ)

Body, self (身 *ŋiŋ)

 Bronze inscription versions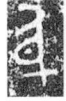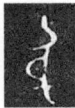

Pregnant, "to become pregnant" (孕 *liŋ-s)

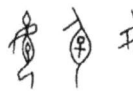

Woman and mother (女 *nraʔ, 母 *məʔ or mˤoʔ)

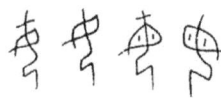

Child (子 *tsəʔ)

give birth," which seemingly has no descendant graph, is directly related to our understanding of early birthing and will be discussed second (second line in chart 2). First, we will examine the connection between the graphs used in later times for birthing and how the Shang use of it as a reference to a recently deceased ancestral spirit may help explain the names of Chu progenitor deities.

The Shang graph of the word later used routinely for "to give birth" 毓 (yu, also written as 育 or 鬻 in the Warring States period) was a Shang term for recently deceased ancestors. It depicted a child emerging out of the woman's body from a side view, sometimes with fluid. Although this word was commonly used in later times in the direct sense of "to give

Chart 2. Shang words related to birthing

To give birth, recently deceased ancestors (毓 *m-quk)

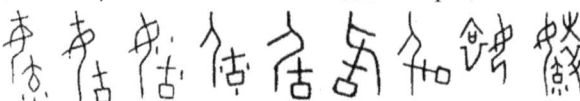

To give birth (no post-Shang versions, read as 冥 *mˤeŋ, 娩 *mror?, or 宛 *ʔor?)

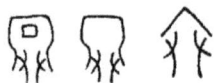

Source, spring (泉 *s-N-ɢʷar)

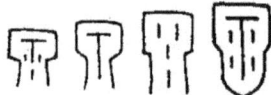

Specially raised sacrificial animal (牢 *r.ŋˤaw)

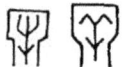

Graphs possibly depicting female and male genitals:
   Abyss (淵 *[ʔ]ʷˤi[ʔ])

   Graph 也 *lAjʔ for pouring vessel 匜 *laj or name 它 *l̥ˤaj

   Birthing   Mystery word with blade and phallus

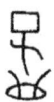

birth," and by extension "to produce," during the Shang period it was primarily reserved to refer to a hierarchy of male and female ancestors dating back several generations. The word could refer to one particular ancestor or to a group such as the Many Yu (*duo yu* 多毓) or the Five Yu (*wu yu* 五毓).[5] A connection between this ancient usage and the later use of the complex graph 鬻 (also meaning "to nourish" and "grain soup") may help explain the use of this latter graph as one of the names for a Chu progenitor. Although there is no oracle bone version of this graph, a very close version with "wood" 木 instead of "grain" 米 in between the sides of a cooking vessel is seen at the top of chart 3 on page 6. This graph was also used as a name, but, because of the fragmented nature of the oracle bone record, we know nothing about it. There are no other examples of similar names until the Warring States period (475–221 BCE). In the Chu bamboo divination texts from Baoshan 包山 (located in modern Hubei), this ancestor's name is written as "birth" (yu 毓, although with a "female" 女 element rather than a 每; the 㐬 element was misunderstood and written as a double 虫 element). In the Xin Cai 新蔡 texts (found in modern Henan), the same name is written slightly differently: the "female" element is replaced with a "divinity" element 示. The Chu materials from these sites are the only evidence preserved of the possible survival of the layered Shang readings of "birth" and "ancestor" during that later period. We now examine the names of the Three Chu Progenitors (san Chu xian 三楚先) listed on the Baoshan and Xin Cai bamboo records and examine their relationship to birthing.[6]

Chu Ancestral Names and the Word for Birth

A quick look at a title or sobriquet commonly applied to Chu royal lineage leaders reveals a possible ancient relationship between genealogy and myth. The title applied to Chu leaders in excavated Warring States Chu materials is written as "Drinker" (䣱, a version of yin 飲 *qəmʔ). A look at the series of yin graphs in chart 3 shows that a human, probably female, element in the more ancient forms of the graph was over the years misunderstood as the element 欠. In transmitted texts, the Chu sobriquet is not Yin but Xiong "Bear" (熊 *C.ɢʷəm, or perhaps a rare word for a sea creature 能 *nˤa).[7] Only in the Xin Cai divination texts does the sobriquet Xiong occur.[8] The Three Chu Progenitors in all Baoshan and some Xin Cai examples are: Lao Tong 老童 "Old Boy," Zhu Rong 祝融 "Invoker Melder," and Yu Yin 毓䣱 "Birth Drinker." In a couple of cases in the Xin Cai list of the three, "Birth Drinker" is replaced with Xue Xiong 穴熊 "Cave Bear." See chart 3 for how they are written in the Baoshan and Xin Cai materials.

In the Chu ju, the father of the baby born with the identifier of Thorn (Chu) was "Xue Yin," a combination of Xue Xiong and Yu Yin, confirming that the two names for some people actually represented one

Chart 3. Chu progenitor names and related graphs

Shang word similar to 鬻 (*m-quk) but with 木 instead of 米:

 Shuowen

Chu ju word for auspicious birth 毓 (*m-quk):

Baoshan and Xin Cai terms for the Three Chu Progenitors 三楚先:

Lao Tong 老童 (*C.rˤuʔ-[d]ˤoŋ) 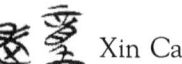 Xin Cai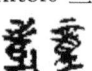

Zhu Rong 祝融 (*[t]uk-luŋ) 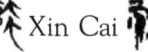 Xin Cai (alternative for Rong*lum)

Yu Yin 妴(鬻)畬(熊) (*m-quk-q(r)[ə]m?) Xin Cai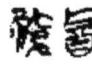

(Xin Cai) Xue Xiong (*[ɢ]ʷˤi[t]-C.ɢʷəm)

Versions of yin (Shang through Warring States periods):

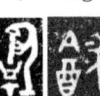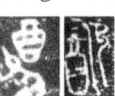

Shang version of the element 欠:

A version of rong from the Late Western Zhou Chu Gongni bell:

Versions of tong from Shang through Warring States periods:

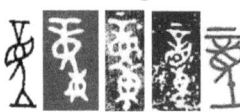

Shang and Xin Cai versions of xiong:

Qin word with "cave" and "toad":   Shang for "toad":

Shang and Western Zhou versions of the 鬲 "vessel" element: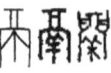

founder god. It seems odd that the scribes and diviners of the Chu religious tradition would not preserve a single name for a deity. If the alternative names were simply the result of phonetic loans, we might understand that the different graphs represented the reality of a variety of scribes attempting to draw upon different oral traditions, how we might imagine the tales of ancient founders were transmitted. However, if we look at the phonetically reconstructed pronunciations of the gods in chart 3, we see a much more complex situation. Each name consists of two syllables and with the exception of Xue, the first syllables all end with rounded vowels and velar finals (*-uʔ or -uk) and the second syllables all end with nasalized finals, mostly velars, two with rounded vowels and two with mid-central slightly rounded vowels (*-oŋ, -uŋ, -əm). If we were going to condense the three gods into a theoretical single, accounting for the dropping of some differences (dropping in some dialects is represented by the brackets) and collapse similarly pronounced phonetics, then we might end up with one or two deities named Ukeng, Dukong, Gukum (or some variant thereof).

The outlier is the name with the preface of Xue 穴 ("cave, hole"). It turns out that the graph *xue* appears in Shang and Western Zhou inscriptions only as a semantic element attached to other graphs, often but not always as a name.[9] To explore the idea that Xue in the Chu names was originally just an attached semantic element to the Xiong, note that in the third and second to last two lines of chart 3 the Shang and Xin Cai versions of the graph for "Bear" are compared with an early Spring and Autumn Qin loan word for "early" (*zao* 早). The Qin word, most likely a loan from the graph "stove" (*zao* 竈), consisted of a "cave" semantic over the "toad" phonetic.[10] Although it is unlikely that the graphs for "toad" and "bear" were in fact confused for each other in antiquity (although there are very few existing examples of either), we use the Qin graph to suggest that Xue was possibly simply part of an older graph for the Chu sobriquet and became detached during the creation of a written tradition by Chu scribes, perhaps even ones unfamiliar with the ancient names or the actual deities. It is unfortunate that there are no Chu religious texts earlier than the fourth century BCE that mention these deities' names.

It is possible that the creation of the names for Lao Tong and Zhu Rong underwent a similar metamorphosis. Very little is known about these deities. Only in one place in the *Shanhaijing* 山海經 are they listed together, and elsewhere they are given a variety of identities and names (see discussion on p. 79).¹¹ It seems then that the transcription of the names of Chu progenitor deities varied according to the different scribes and traditions. If we examine the graphs that make up the names and look at the evolution of these graphs from the Shang through the Warring States periods (see the central section of chart 3), we can see where confusion might be possible, particularly with regard to the "vessel" elements, which seem to vacillate between variations of 鬲 and 酉 types, some with the phonetics 今 (*[k]r[ə]m) (for yin, an element also possibly confused with xue) and some with a double "insect" 虫 phonetic (*C.lruŋ) (for Baoshan and Xin Cai versions of Rong and Yu). Scholar Li Jiahao 李家浩 has shown that the double "insect" element was really a misunderstanding of the simplified graph for yu "birth," which was originally depicted with an upside-down infant with fluid underneath (㐬 *ru) (see the second line in chart 3 for the Chu ju version of "to give birth").¹² The graph for Rong in Zhu Rong presumably had a double "vessel" element as well (something that could possibly have been confused with versions of Tong in the name Lao Tong). Other elements—such as the "female" 女, "divinity" 示, "releasing one's breath" 欠, and "insect"—also seem to get confused. Although it is hard to imagine that Chu ritual officers would rely only on a written tradition for tales of their gods, I suspect that the names of old gods (or of a single god) were adapted to new purposes. For example, we see Zhu Rong defined by Han times as a god associated with the management of the cosmic process of Fire (with links to the supernatural influences of Mars and the South). Yu Xiong, on the other hand, was provided a distinguished lineage beginning with his work for the Zhou founder King Wen 文王. There are no pre-Han texts with these associations.

The complex form of the graph used for the deity's name Yu 鬻 in transmitted genealogies for the Chu clearly also still carried the meaning of "birth" in the Warring States time. We see it used in the third-century BCE Fangmatan 放馬灘 Day Book, discovered in Gansu Province, to refer to healthy deliveries by animals and birds when they listened to the right music:¹³

> 毛者孕鬻, 胎生者不殰, 而卵生者不殈, 則樂之道歸焉耳.
> The mammals get pregnant and give birth (yu), the fetuses will not be stillborn (or miscarried) and, as for those who give birth with eggs, they will not be infertile (or broken), due to (maintaining the proper) Way of Music.

The Han-period *Shuowen* 說文 dictionary (*Explicated Patterns*, by Xu Shen 許慎, 58–147 CE) preserves on old version of the graph (see chart 3, top line) that included the graph for "to give birth" 毓 in place of the common Han use of the "grain" 米 element (clearly a simplification or complete misreading of the old graph). The tall sides of the "vessel" (evident in a Shang version) are preserved in archaic variants 鬻 and 鬵. It is possible that aspects of an ancient version of a word for birth with an outer enclosure (see chart 2, second series) were misread over time as a "cave" element.

The association of the Chu ur-god (or gods) with birth may be simply a matter of phonetic loan and not, as suggested earlier, the perpetuation of an old Shang term for the hierarchy of recently deceased ancestors. The names of elite Chu males associated with the ruling family included the sobriquet "Drinker" or "Bear" (obvious phonetic loans). We do not know if they received these titles at birth; if they had to earn them; or if, perhaps like the Shang use of the posthumous title "god" (*di* 帝), they were added only after death.

A Lost Word for Birth

The Shang commonly used a graphic and intimate image to represent the verb "to give birth" especially as applied to elite females (see chart 2, second line). The Shang graph shows what might be an enclosure or perhaps even a symbolic womb. Inside the enclosure was a small square depicting perhaps the crowning baby head and two hands reaching to hold on to it. Support for this idea is found in the graph for "child," marking the head with the same type of square form. The ancient graph for "to give birth" does not emphasize the whole female body or the amniotic fluids coming out of it (as in *yu*, chart 2, first line, discussed on p. 3). Instead we see two hands reaching into the enclosure that suggest technical intervention. Most births recorded were royal family events and most likely involved birthing professionals, such as midwives, who in the earliest transmitted records also acted as shamans (*wu* 巫). The outer form, whether also indicating a special enclosure or even the womb, is found in a few other ancient graphs and may have been associated with earthly fluids and the provision of sacred animals for ancestral sacrifices.[14]

Similar Shang oracle bone graphs suggest cognate concepts with the ideas of enclosures that produce things, such as water or animals raised especially for sacrifice. We see that the Shang graph for "source, spring" (*quan* 泉) with water and a "divinity" 示 semantic inside the same graphic element was associated with a womb above (see chart 2, third line). The idea of an enclosure is repeated in the word for a specially raised sacrificial animal (*lao* 牢) (chart 2, fourth line). Inside the enclosure, we see a graph representing a bovid or buffalo (*niu* 牛). Variant versions included different animals such as goats or pigs.[15] The ancient words for "source, spring, and sacrificial animal" were close in pronunciation and may have been related words. The only other Shang graphic form that was graphically close was possibly ancestral to that for "cave" (*xue* 穴), but there barely exists any record of its use other than as an added sematic element to names. Also, as we noted previously, *xue* was not close in its archaic pronunciation.

The descendant graph and the underlying word for the Shang verb "to give birth" remain a mystery.[16] Scholars have suggested that the image of the graph for "to give birth" was somewhat like Warring States–period versions of a word for "darkness" *ming* 冥 (*mˤeŋ), but it must be read as "to give birth," *mian* 娩 (*mror? or mran?).[17] The choice of *ming* was influenced by the shape of the graph and by the Han use of "obscure darkness" (*mingming*) to describe the place where humans were conceived and out of which they emerged in birth, an image that was used in early Daoist texts.[18] Unfortunately, a clear phonetic lineage from the Shang cluster of related graphs (*ŋʷar, s-N-ɢʷar, r.ŋˤaw) cannot be easily connected to the later word "to give birth" *yu* 毓 (*m-quk) or to any of the Chu progenitors' names. However, Yu Xiong is linked in myth in the late Warring States period with the creator couple Fuxi 伏羲 and Nüwa 女媧—discussed later—and the pronunciation of their names was closer to the Shang cluster (see chart 6). Nevertheless, we must keep in mind that the pronunciation of words and their usage inevitably changed dramatically over the millennium of time that passed between the Shang and the Warring States periods (for which the phonetic reconstruction system we are using can be considered most valid). And, indeed, new vocabulary replaced old.

In the Warring States period, such as in the case of our Chu text, the *Chu ju*, the word for birth (*yu* 毓) was used as the progenitor's name in the Baoshan text and for the verb for the (auspicious) birth of the first set of twins born to the descended god-king Ji Lian 季連. Another word used for birthing in the text was the more common and generic term *sheng* 生, which was originally associated with spring growth in the natural (versus the human) sphere. First, referring to the natural generation of vegetative or astral forms, in Warring States philosophical discourse, it was applied abstractly to when one phenomenon could "give rise to" (*sheng*) another phenomenon and, in genealogical narratives, when one male ancestor could "generate" (*sheng*) male descendants.[19] This allowed genealogical narratives to suppress historical acknowledgment of the female role in social reproduction, which was represented by the word *yu*. We will discuss the genealogical narratives in chapter 5.

Suggestive Images

Since textual records were dominated by the need for social reproduction of the patriarchy and male scribes, it is difficult to recover a sense of women's experience with childbirth from texts. Images from Neolithic through Han material culture can be suggestive. In the Neolithic, we have symbolic images on pottery, sculptures of pregnant women, and a phallus made of clay—all hinting at a concern with fertility.

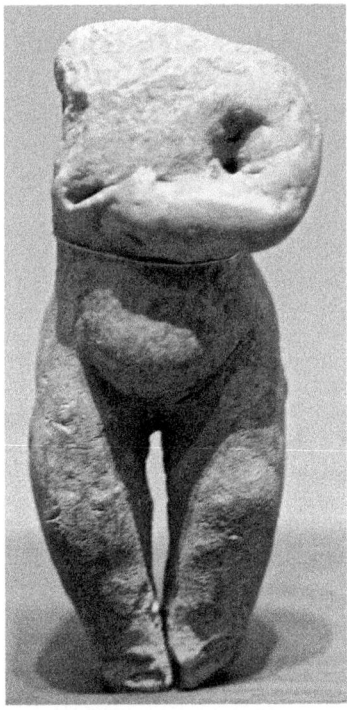

Figure 1. Hongshan sculpture of a pregnant body, excavated in 1982 from Dongshanzui, Kazuo, Chaoyang City, Liaoning Province 遼寧省朝陽市喀左東山嘴. National Museum of China. Photo by Tian Shuai.

12 / Birth in Ancient China

The Hongshan culture, of the fifth through third millennia BCE, located far to the northeast of what would be the Chinese heartland area, clearly worshipped the pregnant female body. There, archaeologists discovered a round shrine filled with statues of naked pregnant women, with obvious breasts and protruding bellies. As we saw from the analysis of the words for birth earlier, the protruding belly, symbol of the enclosure within which the fetus generates, represented "self" and the full human body. The reproductive capability of women ensured a key role in ancient society, one that would cause anxiety once patriarchal hierarchies and lineage politics began to form during the late Neolithic period. The sculptures in the shrine dedicated to the female body were likely used for fertility worship. Also from this culture came many bracelet-like jades of encircled dragon figures. Many of these found their way into the heartland Neolithic cultures, but no other versions of the shrine have been found.[20] Nor seemingly did the custom for the voluptuous depiction of sculpted naked female bodies spread.

In a roughly contemporary culture called Banpo 半坡, farther south in modern Shaanxi, and closer to the heartland where politicized hierarchies first became evident, we find abstract images that may be symbolic vulvas giving birth. Painted on the sides of ceramic bowls, vulva-like triangles sometimes also depicted a baby's face emerging from

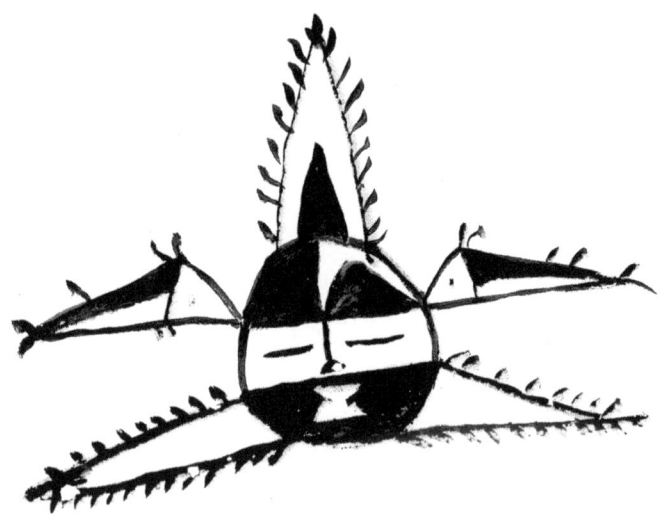

Figure 2. Banpo pottery bowl paintings with baby faces. Drawing by C. A. Cook (adapted from photographs by Cook taken at the Banpo Museum, Shaanxi Province, and by Tian Shuai at the National Museum of China).

the middle triangle shape. Sometimes fish were drawn as well. Fish in much later times were associated with fertility, and in other ancient cultures they were considered phallic. Not all scholars agree that such paintings represented birth images or that the bowl was used in fertility rituals. Some scholars suggest that the face was not that of a baby but instead a representation of a mask worn by a shaman. Of course, without written records from the Neolithic, we cannot be sure. Ceramic phalluses have been found at Neolithic sites in northern China suggesting early fertility rituals.[21] Ceramic vessels with male-female body images have also been discovered (see figure 3), suggesting a particular power linked to hermaphroditic imagery.

The fertility of Fu Hao 婦好, a wife of Shang king Wu Ding 武丁 (ca. 1250–1192 BCE), was obviously important as many oracle bone birthing records concern her. Objects found in her tomb may also be

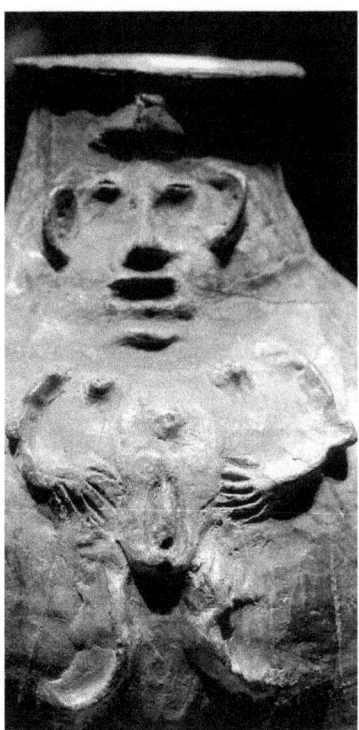

Figure 3. Possible fertility symbolism on a Neolithic pot excavated in 1974 from a Liuwan, Leduxian, Qinghai Province 青海省樂都縣柳灣 site. National Museum of China. Photo by Tian Shuai.

related to her reproductive role. Hand-sized jade amulets depicted male and female symbolism on reverse sides and may have been carried or used in prayer. One is bird-shaped with a phallus engraved on its chest on one side and a "cowry shell"—possibly symbolic of a vulva—form on the other. The other jade amulet was more overt; it depicted a naked girl on one side with a naked boy on the other. They are both wearing antlers, which according to scholars was a likely fertility symbol.[22]

A square caldron (*ding*) placed in Fu Hao's tomb was also cast with antler symbolism inside and out. Antlers were regular features in the Shang period, and later iconography and may have signified multiple meanings associated with death and rebirth, much in the way that snakes, cicadas, and other figures from the animal world do that shed skins, regrow appendages, or undergo metamorphosis.

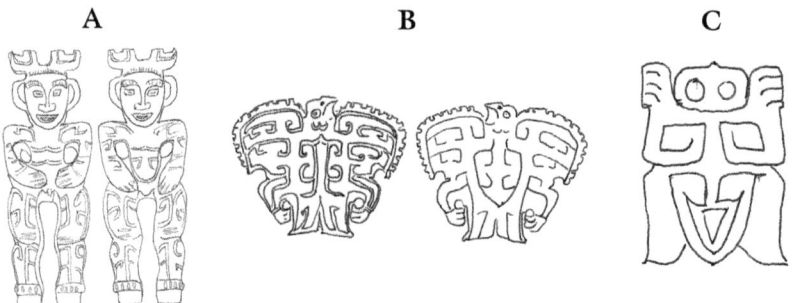

Figure 4. Fu Hao jade amulets with possible fertility symbolism (A, B, and C). Drawings by C. A. Cook (adapted from Zhongguo sheke xueyuan kaogu yanjiusuo 1994, figs. 202.3, 204.5, 205.3). A and B show both sides of the amulets.

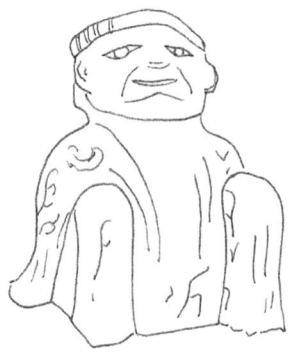

Figure 5. Jade figurine of a woman in a birthing position from Fu Hao's tomb. Drawing by C. A. Cook (adapted from Zhongguo sheke xueyuan kaogu yanjiusuo 1994, fig. 201.1).

We see too some evidence of the "sacred display" of female genitalia—an expression of female power over fertility (documented by Miriam Dexter and Victor Mair for Eurasia) in a small stone figurine leaning backward as well as in other figures.[23] Although we can only speculate on the function of the many figurines, both animal and human, in Fu Hao's tomb, the concern over her fertility expressed in the oracle bones provides a suggestive context. The fact that these items were placed in her tomb suggests an ongoing concern with her role as an ancestor in social reproduction after death.

The tiny jade figurines in her tomb include images of women carved out of jade or stone with highly decorated bodies, often in kneeling positions, perhaps representing subservience or respect. Besides the engravings on their bodies that marked clothing lines and tattoos, they sported headgear and sashes that flew out backward like wing feathers or tail fins, suggesting a magical function. The tomb also contained a giant bronze tripod dedicated to an ancestress "mother."[24] On the handle, the mouths of two tigers (or one "split" tiger) form what could be a symbolic birth opening, out of which a small head appears. Late Shang–period bronze sacrificial vessels in the shape of tigers (with their bodies covered with tattoos of snakes and birds) appear with baby-like humans standing in the tigers' arms and with the human heads in the tigers' mouths. Does this represent sacrifice, birth, death, or all the aforementioned? We can only speculate.

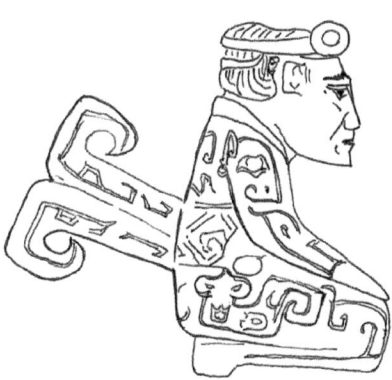

Figure 6. Jade figurine of a woman with tattoos and a bird tail from Fu Hao's tomb. Drawing by C. A. Cook (adapted from Zhongguo sheke xueyuan kaogu yanjiusuo 1994, fig. 200.1).

16 / Birth in Ancient China

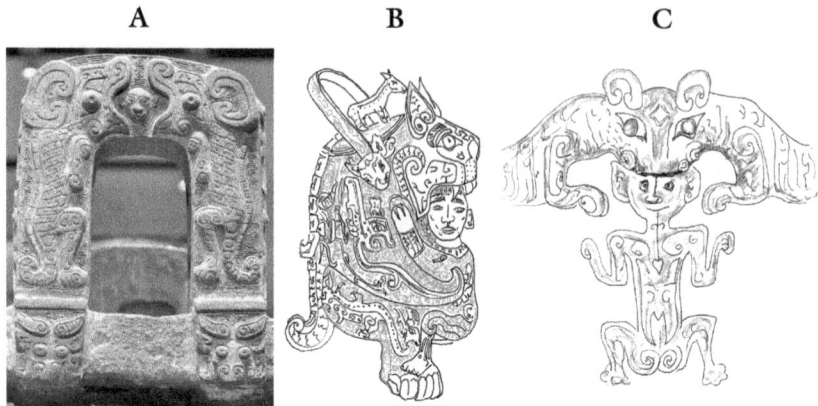

Figure 7. Humans in the mouths of tigers, images from bronzes (A, B, and C).
A. handle decor on a large caldron vessel dedicated to the cult of Royal Mother Wu 后母戊 excavated from Anyang in the 1930s, presently in the National Museum of China. Photo by Tian Shuai.
B. Drawing of Shang *you* vessels found in the Sumitomo Collection in Sen-oku Museum (Kyoto) and in Cernuschi Museum (Paris). Drawing by C. A. Cook (adapted from the Shandong Museum website version of an image from the Shaanxi sheng wenwuju Han Tang wang).
C. Decor from a Shang *zun* vessel in Anhui Museum. Drawing by C. A. Cook (adapted from a photograph on http://blog.sina.com.cn/s/blog_6987f00c0102wdrc.html).

Of interest to our reading of the "split" bodies of mothers from the Chu text is the fact that to show both sides of the tiger mother of the infant, the image was created in split-body form, suggesting an ancient conception of splitting and the birth of an heir. An axe-head dedicated to Fu Hao repeats the motif of the head emerging out of the split tiger mouth. Axes were typically used for cutting off the heads of sacrificial victims, suggesting again a possible connection between the portals of life and death. This shape, besides reminding us of the Shang word for female birthing, is also somewhat like that of the sacred 亞 shape, which Sarah Allan has identified with the shape of the Shang royal tomb, the shape of the tortoise plastron used in divination, and the image of the cosmic diagram of the Four Regions or directions (*sifang* 四方).[25]

Since late Shang bronze inscriptions clearly specify that the vessels were used in the worship of human spirits (fathers, mothers, ancestors), imagery of faces on the sides of vessels, on the vessel handles, or on axe heads (some shown emerging out of enclosures) may be associated with fertility and lineage reproduction. Many of the faces are mask-like with attendant animal pieces as part of their composition, suggesting the performance of shamanistic rituals involving symbolic transformation and communion with the spirit world.[26] In fact such imagery could be multivalent, with the baby or person representing the shaman in transition between the worlds of life and death. The fetal nature of this form, with bent limbs and curling fingers and toes, is particularly obvious in examples where the form emerges either head or feet first out of the mouths of tigers. Their half-animal forms suggest transition between animal and human, a physical metamorphosis suggestive of the times just before birth and after death, or even of a child versus an adult in the later Confucian ideology that a human must be educated to distinguish him- or herself from the more primitive animal state. During the late Shang and into the subsequent Zhou periods, fetal forms were joined with bird instead of tiger imagery and carved into hand-sized amulets of jade that could be worn.

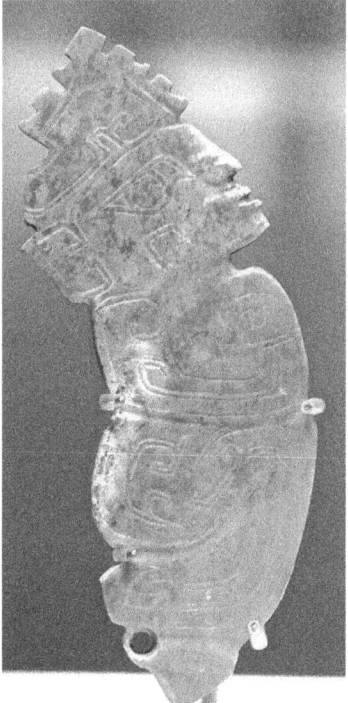

Figure 8. Jade amulet with a fetal-like birdman from the Fu Hao tomb site. National Museum of China. Photo by Tian Shuai.

In much later times, there seems to have been a symbolic connection between the pollution of birth and the pollution of death and the purification and mortuary rituals used to mitigate the negative effects of the contamination.[27] Birth seems to have symbolized the emergence from a state that was equivalent to death. The connections between death, birth, and communication with the spirit world suggest the beginnings of the later Daoist idea of the "mother" as a portal between the states of life and death (an image explored in chapter 3). Shang-period images of fetal-like forms emerging from/going into tiger mouths on bronze vessels suggest a connection between sacrifices to ancestors and fertility prayers. This is particularly true for the variations of this form in which the front of the body is marked by a symbolic cicada body, representing perhaps a vulva-like form and eternal life.[28]

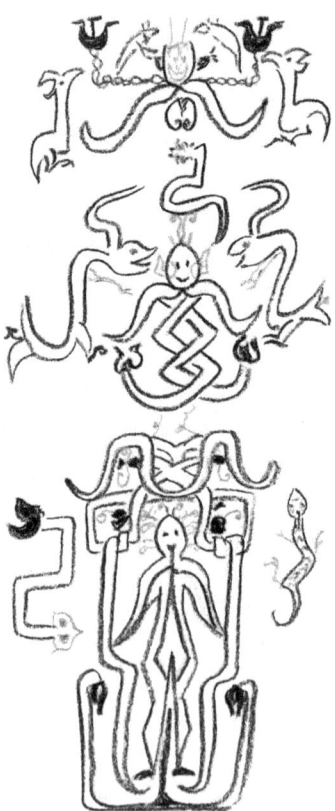

Figure 9. Figures with split bodies found on the inner coffin of Zeng Hou Yi (d. 443 BCE). Drawing by C. A. Cook (adapted from Hubei sheng bowuguan 1989, vol. 2, fig. 11.4, and Hubei sheng bowuguan 1991, figs. 281, 282, 284).

We find a curious extension of this type of form in the supernatural forms drawn outside the coffin of a Lord Yi of Zeng (who died in 443 BCE), an ally of the Chu royal family. The application of fertility symbols to mortuary architecture continues into the Han period, where we find tomb gateways marked with engravings of the intertwined snake-like dragon bodies of the creator god and goddess Fuxi 伏羲 and Nüwa 女媧. These figures (also found as coffin decor and on jades) symbolize the primal couple and are first mentioned in the Chu Silk Manuscript, dating to around the same time as the *Chu ju*. The fact that they would appear on tomb doors confirms their symbolic role as controlling the portal between life and death.

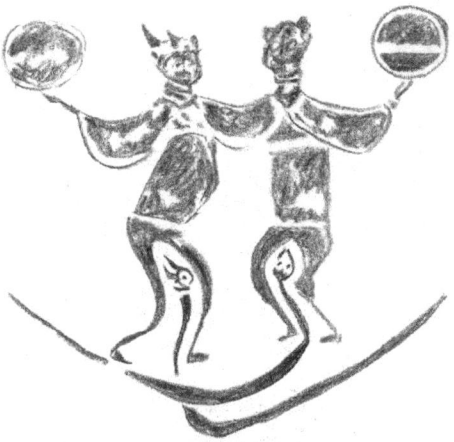

Figure 10. Fuxi and Nüwa with snake tails and holding the sun and moon, from a Han stone sarcophagus, excavated in Chongqing, Sichuan, in 1980. Presently in the Chongqing National Sanxia Museum. Drawing by C. A. Cook (adapted from Luo Erhu 2002, 136).

2

Controlling Reproduction
Fertility Prayers

Control over the human reproductive process has always been key to the evolution of civilization, its sense of history, and identity. While we have no knowledge of the herbs or other physical means for controlling fertility in remote antiquity, the artistic motifs examined previously and early records suggest a concern with fertility and a desire to control the outcome of the female birthing experience. Texts documenting the prayers, divinations, and sacrifices from the Shang up through early imperial times reflect continued and evolving, primarily religious, methods for acquiring heirs who were charged with remembering the past.

The earliest written prayers are preserved on Shang oracle bones. Although the records on the oracle bones are fragmented and provide few complete samples, we do have preserved from the Wu Ding period a complete prayer concerning the fertility of his wife Fu Hao as well as the king's interpretation of a possibly auspicious response from the cracking of the bone. In *Jiaguwen heji* (bone number 94, front), we find:[1]

> 辛丑卜殼貞: 婦好有子, 二月.
> 辛丑卜亘貞; 王占曰: 好其有子, 禦.
> Divining on a Xinchou day (day thirty-eight of the sixty-day ritual calendar), Que prognosticated: "Fu Hao will be with child in the second month."
> Divining on a Xinchou day, Xuan prognosticated. The king read the cracks and pronounced, "Hao will perhaps be with child. Perform a (protective) exorcism."

Peng Bangjiong 彭邦炯 claims that the oracle bone terms "seeking to be with child" (*qiu sheng* 求生) versus "receiving a pregnancy" (*shou sheng* 受生) involved separate sets of prayers.[2] In the former category are inscriptions asking whether a birth might occur (*wang* 亡 or *wu/you sheng* 无/有生). Sacrifices and prayers for fertility were made to spirits, which scholar Hu Houxuan has suggested might be early versions of the Gaomei–style rituals documented in later texts and discussed on pp. 31ff.[3] From divinations seeking children for the king, specific female ancestors were often the objects of prayer.[4] Peng suggests that once the women began to show symptoms of pregnancy, diviners had to confirm that the symptoms were in fact due to pregnancy, and then whether the pregnancy would come to term. For example, in *Heji* 13925 (front side of the bone):[5]

丁酉卜賓貞: 婦好有受生.
Divining on Dingyou day, Bin prognosticates: "Fu Hao will have received (the divine intervention) to give birth."

Another way to query this issue was to ask if "there would be pregnancy" (*you yun* 有孕) or "would there be children" (*you zi* 有子) (Peng tries to claim that the term *shou sheng* was only used for the first trimester and *you yun* and *you zi* for the next, but there is no way to prove this).[6] The use of the word "to have, to possess" (*you*) by the fourth century BCE had taken on a Daoist meaning of "having things" or "forms," in other words existence versus nonexistence (a concept discussed in terms of "motherhood" in the next chapter). The Shang idea of "receiving" the ability to give birth suggests that pregnancy was seen as a divine gift associated with their ancestral spirits. This reflects the role of the female ancestor spirits and, in later examples, the role of other deities, gods or Di.[7]

Peng notes one unusual oracle bone record that he feels must belong in the category of worrying if there will or will not be a child: "Shaman Mei catches a child" 巫妹獲子.[8] From our analysis of the words for "giving birth" in the previous chapter, we suggest that, in fact, the "catching" of a child may have been literal. Not only did the record wish that "catching a child" would be possible, but it also documents that shamans served as midwives. This fits well with the ancient Shang graph for "to give birth" and with the *Chu ju* birth record discussed in chapter 5.

Zhou Fertility Prayers in Bronze Inscriptions

Zhou society is typically defined as structured according to a *zongfa* 宗法 model. This model is shaped somewhat like a tree root system, in which a central tap root represented by the original founding ancestor's lineage shrine (*zong*) has innumerable collateral root systems that branch off from the central root but then create their own centralized systems. In this idealized system, the male patriarch that heads each system would have a series of sons, the eldest of which would take over the patriarch's position eventually, and the younger sons would then start their own collateral branch systems with their own branch shrines. Clearly, fertility would be a chief concern to the continuation of all branches of the lineage. We see this concern reflected in the prayers preserved in transmitted texts and in the inscriptions on bronze vessels used to present sacrifices to the ancestral spirits at the lineage shrines. For example, we see in the late Western Zhou–period Liangqi *ding* 梁其鼎 (a type of caldron for meat offerings):[9]

> 梁其作尊鼎, 用享孝于皇祖考, 用祈多福, 眉壽無疆,
> 畯臣天子, 其百子千孫, 其萬年無疆, 其子子孫孫永寶用。
> Liangqi made a caldron to express reverence and to present offerings to (the spirits of his) Brilliant Ancestor and Deceased Father and to pray for much good fortune, long life without end, to be able to serve the Son of Heaven, and perhaps one hundred sons and one thousand grandsons; May he (live) ten thousand years without limit and have sons of sons and grandsons of grandsons eternally treasure and use (this caldron to present offerings).

For the Zhou people, ancestral spirits were the lineage protectors. Elites like Liangqi prayed to the ancestors to get what they wanted. So, he prayed to his powerful ancestors as well as his deceased father—the spirit most invested in his son's success—for wealth, long life, career success, and an endless stream of descendants (who would worship him just like he did his own ancestral spirits). We find similar prayers recorded on many inscriptions. On three inscriptions dated to the Middle Western Zhou period, for example, we find the vessels used for prayers for wealth, long life, and fertility. The Guai Bo *gui* 乖伯簋 (tureen for grain and other dishes) has:[10]

用祈屯祿, 永命, 魯壽, 子孫
Use it to pray for accumulated salary, eternal life allotment, a prosperous long life, and descendants.

The Zuojue wenzu *fangzun* 作厥文祖方尊 (a square alcohol storage vessel) has:[11]

其用匄永福, 萬年, 子孫.
May it be used for seeking eternal good fortune, ten thousand years of life, and descendants.

We find these same concerns expressed to ancestor spirits on Late Western Zhou inscriptions. The Liusheng *xu* 翏生盨 (another type of tureen),[12] for example, records Liusheng's contribution to the Zhou state—his accompaniment of the king on a military campaign against the rebellious southeastern peoples called the Huaiyi 淮夷. He follows this record with his prayer to his ancestors:

翏生眔大妘其百男, 百女, 千孫, 其萬年眉壽.
May Liusheng and Dayun (his wife) have one hundred boys, one hundred girls, and one thousand grandsons. May they have ten thousand years of extended long life.

Liusheng's prayer for his wife to have hundreds of progeny and thousands of descendants is a classic Zhou fertility prayer. Most bronze inscriptions included a section for invoking blessings, and these requests reflect the social concerns of the people: wealth, long life, career success, and abundant fertility. For a lineage to continue and a specific society to continue, they relied on descendants to replicate the social structures and the ancestors to protect them.[13]

The addition of prayers at the end of bronze inscriptions did not become common until around the ninth century BCE. Shang and even most Early Western Zhou–period inscriptions (mid-eleventh through mid-tenth centuries BCE) did not include the common prayer for "sons of sons and grandsons of grandsons to eternally treasure (or protect) and use (the vessel)" (*zizi sunsun yong bao yong* 子子孫孫永寶/保用), although it is likely that sacrifices to the ancestors did involve prayers for all social issues, including fertility. The idea of endless lines of descendants is explained later in the "Tang wen" 湯問 chapter of the transmitted text

Liezi 列子 (compiled in the fourth century CE out of earlier sources):¹⁴

> 子又生孫, 孫又生子, 子又有子, 子又有孫, 子子孫孫, 無窮匱也.
> The son will produce a grandson, and then the grandson will produce a son, and that son has a son, who in turn has a grandson; so, sons of sons and grandsons of grandsons means to continue on endlessly.

While the prayer does not directly ask for female fertility from the ancestors, it does show the Zhou concern for social reproduction through an abundance of descendants.

This concern continued after the fall of the Zhou hegemony into the Eastern Zhou period, also known as the Spring and Autumn and Warring States periods—a time of war and social instability. We find more specific fertility prayers, some that request "boys and girls without limit" (*nannüwuqi* 男女無期), "the proliferation of sons and grandsons" (*zisun fanchang* 子孫蕃昌), or "let there be one hundred such boys" (*bei bai sinan* 卑百斯男).¹⁵ The Gong Dian *pan* 公典盤 (a basin for ablution), excavated from a Spring and Autumn–period tomb in Changqing 長清, Shandong, had the following inscription:¹⁶

> 郜子姜首及郜, 公典為其盥盤, 用祈眉壽難老, 室家是保, 它它熙熙, 男女無期, 于終有卒, 子子孫孫永保用之, 不用勿出.
> When Jiang Shou (wife) of the Scion of Shi went (in marriage) to Shi, Dian the Patriarch (of Shi) made a washing basin for her, so that she may pray for extended long life with no aging, for protection for her home; extensively and splendidly¹⁷ (may she have) limitless boy and girl children and be endlessly fertile, so sons of sons and grandsons of grandsons will eternally protect and use it (the vessel). When not in use do not bring it out.

From this inscription, we know that a Jiang-lineage woman married into the Shi state household and that the ruler of it commemorated the marriage with an inscribed bronze basin specifically used to pray for blessings and reproductive fertility from the ancestral spirits. During the Spring and Autumn, a time of increasing political conflict, we find the otherwise unusual acknowledgment that both male and female children are necessary for social reproduction. We see this again in a

Late Spring and Autumn–period inscription on the Qi Hou *dui* 齊侯敦 (a grain vessel):[18]

> 齊侯作媵寬虞孟姜善敦, 用祈眉壽, 萬年無疆,
> 它它熙熙, 男女無期, 子子孫孫永保用之.
> The Lord of Qi made a dowry vessel *dui* for the Jiang-lineage woman who got married in a place named Kuanyu, so that she may pray for extended long life, ten thousand years without limit, extensively and splendidly (may she have) limitless boy and girl children, so sons of sons and grandsons of grandsons will eternally protect and use it (the vessel).

We find the same rhetorical formulas on the Qing Shu *yi* 慶叔匜 (a pouring vessel) of the same time period:[19]

> 慶叔作媵子孟姜盥匜, 其眉壽萬年, 永保其身,
> 它它熙熙, 男女無期, 子子孫孫永保用之.
> The Secondary Son of Qing made a washing basin as a dowry vessel for the Jiang-lineage woman (wife) of the Scion. May she have extended long life, ten thousand years, eternal protection over her body, extensively and splendidly (may she have) limitless boys and girls, so sons of sons and grandsons of grandsons will eternally protect and use it.

The previous three bronze inscriptions are all dowry inscriptions for Qi women made to commemorate their marriages to regional lords. Clearly, the royal houses valued females for their physical roles in continuing the family line. We might imagine that the vessels, no matter whether for bathing or holding grain or alcohol during the ceremonies for the ancestral spirits, acted like the women's bodies themselves as mediums between the spirit world and human, providing communal continuity over time and space.

The recently discovered Baozi *ding* 鮑子鼎 (a caldron for meat offerings) dating to the same time period repeats many of the same concerns but with an added twist:[20]

> 鮑子作媵仲匋姒, 其獲皇男子, 勿有闌已, 它它熙熙, 男女無期,
> 仲匋姒及子思, 其壽君毋死, 保而兄弟, 子子孫孫永保用.
> Baozi made a dowry vessel for a Si-lineage woman of Middle Son Tao. May she have supreme boy children, not ever stop-

ping, extensively and splendidly (may she have) limitless boys and girls. May the Si-woman of Middle Son Tao when she comes to Scion Si bring long life to the Lord with no death and (cause the spirits) to protect the elder and younger brothers, so sons of sons and grandsons of grandsons will eternally protect and use it (the vessel).

The focus of the social reproduction in this inscription moves from just the woman's requirement to produce boys and girls to the need to produce especially fine boys, heirs who, like the later superior men, the *junzi* 君子, could be specially trained for roles in government.

We see also that fertility prayers were part of marriage ceremony records inscribed into a washing basin and alcohol container in the southeastern state of Wu during the sixth century BCE. In 1955, archaeologists discovered the tomb of Lord Shen of Cai 蔡侯申 (identified by many scholars as Lord Zhao of Cai 蔡昭侯, r. 519–491 BCE, or the earlier Lord Ping of Cai 蔡平侯, r. 522–530) in Shouxian, Anhui Province. The tomb had been plundered, but besides vessels belonging to Lord Shen, there were also prominently displayed a round *jian*-basin with a smaller round *fou* 缶 (alcohol storage jar) inside sent as part of a dowry for a younger Ji-lineage 姬 woman who was a princess in King Guang of Wu's court.[21] In the northwestern corner of the tomb was another complete set of food, alcohol, and cooking and serving dowry vessels for Cai Zhao Hou Shen's eldest daughter (or perhaps sister) to marry a king of Wu. Scholars date the vessels to 519 BCE, the first year of Cai Zhao Hou Shen's rule according to the *Shiji* 史記 (*Records of the Historian*), and suggest that the intended groom was Wu king Guang's cousin, Liao 僚, whom Guang murdered in 515 BCE to take up the throne himself.[22] The inscription is longer than a simple dowry inscription, perhaps recording details of the ceremony itself:

元年正月初吉辛亥，蔡侯申虔恭大命，上下陟否（敷?），[23] 祗敬不惕（易），肇差（佐）天子. 用詐（作）大孟姬媵（滕）彝盤. 禋享是以祗盟（明）嘗啻（禘），祐受母已，齋叚（嘏）整肅，類文王母，穆穆亹亹，恩（聰）害（吾＞御）[24] 訢（慎）[25] 昜（揚），威義（儀）遊遊，[26] 靈頌（容）託（度）商（章），康諧龢好，敬配吳王. 不諱（違）考壽，子孫蕃昌，永保用之，終歲無疆. It was in the first year, first month, Early auspicious (*chuji*), on Xinhai day [no. 48], that Lord Shen of Cai paid his respects to the Great Mandate, to those above and below, promoting (the worthy) and spreading (the mandate). He has acted with sincere respect making no changes (in his loyalties): he was an aid to the Son of Heaven. He takes this opportunity to make for his eldest daughter of the Ji lineage a metal basin for her dowry sacrificial vessels to present (to the spirits) pure ale in mortuary feasts and hence to pay her respects to the Earth, for the luminous rites, for the autumnal tasting rites, and the annual ancestral sacrifices and so as to receive divine aid without end. In fasting and paying her respects, she is upright and serious, measuring herself according to King Wen's mother: grave, so grave; diligent, so diligent; intelligent, supreme, careful, praiseworthy, her Awesome Decorum is performed in a leisurely sauntering manner, and with a numinous look and lovely expression, creating peace, unity, harmony, and affection with which she expresses her respectful nature to become the mate for the king of Wu. Do not behave in a way that violates your ability to live long so that your sons and grandsons are abundant and so as to eternally protect and use (the vessels), and (may your) years be without end.

The prayers to the ancestors as well as to the Earth followed the presentation of the bride. They document for the ancestors her fine qualities and how she measures up to the idealized tradition of Zhou founder King Wen's mother. Her performance of "Awesome Decorum," a musical performance for displaying *de* documented on many bronze inscriptions of men was also especially fine—although notably, the word *de* was not used in her case. Her fertility is implied in her numinous complexion but reinforced with prayers to the ancestors who watched her performance and would share in the joyous ceremony through the sacrificial alcohol and food. The fact that these vessels were originally intended for ancestral shrine sacrifices suggests that once the prayers were cast, they were theoretically repeated to the ancestors whenever the vessels were used in sacrifices. The focus on producing males reflects the political anxiety for survival by the states of Cai and Wu in the wars with the Chu to their southwest.

The emphasis on producing males is also found on an unusually long bell inscription from Late Spring and Autumn Qi. Unlike the dowry vessels used to present offerings to the spirits, this set of bells was produced for a man who was being rewarded by his ruler for military success (a symbol of his *de*). Only in the last section in which he eulogizes his male and female ancestors does he add the prayer for long life, wealth, protection, and the power "to have one hundred *such* boys" (*bi bai si nan* 俾百斯男), presumably referring to boys *just as* glorious as his ancestors. The role of his wife is referred to only obliquely with the use of a causative "to make" (*bi* 俾), yet he referred directly to his father and mother by name in his praise song of his personal history. His wife would not count as a "mother" in the lineage until she had produced an heir.[27]

The prayers for personal and lineage welfare were sent to the ancestors through the supernatural agency of the shiny vessels used in the sacrifices to communicate and entertain the ancestral spirits with food, alcohol, and music. The fragrances and sounds transmitted the prayers upward. The repeated formulaic nature of these prayers placed at the end of inscriptions reflects their popularity over time and the general concern for social continuity.

A Warring States Prayer Preserved on Bamboo Strips

Fertility prayers and rituals performed to spirits other than ancestors are evident in transmitted and bamboo texts after the Spring and Autumn. In this section, we examine rites performed out in the wild. We saw earlier in the long inscription recording the presentation of the bride during a wedding ceremony that the bride was praised for emulating the founder king of Zhou's mother, King Wen's mother 文王母, and that she also gave offerings to the Earth. Since early times there occurred worship of spirits from "above and below" (*shangxia* 上下). By the late fourth century BCE, we know that the natural agencies of Heaven and Earth, like Yang and Yin, were considered formative cosmic influences. Up above was the Sky god(s), Tian 天 ("Heaven") or Shangdi 上帝 ("High God"), master reinforcer of the patriarchy.[28] Down below were gods that reigned over wild and built spaces. They were associated with mountains, fields, trees, rivers, and residences. Some mountain gods were the prehistoric sage Di 帝, who had "descended" from Tian. Lords of the Earth (*dizhu* 地主) were worshipped inside and outside built spaces. It is unclear which if any of the natural spirits were female or, at least, Yin versions of Yang spirits (the clear association of gender with Yin and Yang cannot be proven until the Han period, 206 BCE–220 CE).[29]

Records of rites including nature spirits and other Di flourished after the Spring and Autumn when scribes were not constrained to worship of the Zhou royal lineage and its ancestors.[30] However, association with the Zhou lineage (Ji 姬) was considered particularly auspicious despite the disintegration of its hegemony over politics and religion during the eighth century BCE. The classic of ancient poetry and song, the *Book of Odes* (*Shijing* 詩經), preserves the ode "Birth of the People" ("Shengmin" 生民),[31] which commemorates the smooth birth of the mythical Zhou founder, an earth and grain god named Hou Ji 后稷. His mother famously prayed to Di (possibly Shangdi) for fertility while performing a dance that symbolized "stepping on Di's toeprint." This famous tale, translated and discussed further on p. 40, is reflected in a prayer found in the *Zigao* 子羔, a Warring States bamboo text preserved in the Shanghai Museum.[32] On strips 12 and 13 we find:

> 后稷之母，有邰氏之女也，游于串咎之內，終[33]見芙攼而薦之，乃見人武，履以祈禱曰：'帝之武尚吏 (使) [子?],[34]是后稷之母也。[35]
> "Hou Ji's mother was a woman of Tai. She was wandering around Chuanjiu when she came upon an *au*-thistle stalk, so she presented it as an offering; she saw a human footprint, so she stepped on it and prayed: 'May Di's toe print make me with child!' And so she became Hou Ji's mother."

Fragments of this tale appear in the transmitted texts, with the oldest reference being the ode "Birth of the People." The following discussion will draw on numerous textual and anthropological resources to uncover the fertility ritual performed by Jiang Yuan, the mother of the Zhou people. In chapter 6 we will further compare the account with that of the mother of the Chu people.

Jiang Yuan became pregnant by stepping on the imprint of Di's toe. This tale is also found in the chapter on the Zhou house in the *Shiji* (the "Zhou benji" 周本紀) with the added detail, similar to the *Zigao* account, that she originated from the household of Tai 邰.[36] The version in the *Book of Odes* did not specify the place where she performed the ritual; the *Shiji* simply says "the wilds" (*ye* 野). The place-name Chuanjiu 串咎 in the *Zigao* version is unknown, and many scholars believe it must be a loan. Ma Chengyuan suggested that it should be read as Chuanze 串澤 "Chuan Swamp," perhaps influenced by the earlier scholarship of Wen Yiduo 聞一多 and Chen Mengjia 陳夢家 regarding the fertility rites performed in the Chu swamp Yunmeng 雲夢.[37] Ma's identification rests on the claim that the word *jiu* 咎 ("afflicted by spiritual blame") was a loan for "swamp" (*ze* 澤); unfortunately, the two words were not very close in pronunciation, *gruʔ versus *lˤrak. Ma felt that such a swamp might have been in the Chuanyi 串夷 territory of western non-Sinitic peoples (mentioned in the *Book of Odes*). Others recommend reading "hill" (*qiu* 丘 *k^{wh}ə) for *jiu*; this was slightly closer in pronunciation but still not a homophone.[38] Whether the site was a swamp or a hill cannot be resolved. Wen Yiduo and Chen Mengjia found evidence for fertility rites at both types of sites. These were called variously as Gao Tang 高唐, Gao Mi 高密, Gaomei 高禖, or Jiaomei 郊禖. The terms seem to stand for three related aspects of the sites: the name of the rites performed there, the name of the sites themselves, and the names of the spirit(s) receiving the rites. The rites are referred to in Warring States, Han, and later texts as "primitive" rites still practiced by childless women. Wen Yiduo and others suggest that many early states had such sites and that the sacred swampland of Yunmeng with a "Shaman Mountain" (Wushan 巫山) may have served as the Chu site. They determined that the rainy mountaintop with a mulberry forest, called Mulberry Mountain 桑山, was the one in the old state of Song 宋 (presumably set up for the Shang descendants after the Zhou takeover in the eleventh century BCE).[39] Textual references provide tantalizing details of transgressive sexual meetings in the wilds as well as rites employing birds, sacrifices, phallic symbols, and mountains.

In the "Yueling" 月令 ("Monthly Ordinances") chapter of the *Ritual Records* (*Liji* 禮記), we see, for example, that "during the middle spring month. . . . the Dark Bird arrives. On the day it arrives, one must sacrifice a large penned animal to/at Gaomei 仲春之月,... 玄鳥至. 至之日, 以太牢祠于高禖." The Dark Bird (or birds) is mentioned also in the *Book of Odes* and the *Chuci* 楚辭 (song texts associated with the state of Chu), northern and southern song collections in the context of the magical birth of the Shang progenitor, Xie 契. This spring festival may have been to celebrate the return of swallows to nest.[40] The *Shanhaijing* 山海經 (*Classic of Mountains and Seas*) chapter on the spirits of the inner region near the sea ("Hainei jing" 海內經) links the Dark Bird to other "dark" (*xuan* 玄) animals that lived on a mountain in the "Gloomy Capital" 幽都, another term for a land of the dead in the *Chuci*.[41] Links between nesting swallows, marriage, and birth of a people are made first by the Han-period commentator Zheng Xuan 鄭玄 (127–200 CE):

燕以施生時來, 巢人堂宇而孚乳, 嫁娶之象也, 媒氏之官以為候. 高辛氏之出, 玄鳥遺卵, 娀簡吞之而生契, 后王以為媒宮嘉祥, 而立其祠焉. 變媒言禖, 神之也.

When the time came for swallows to give birth, they built nests in buildings to nurse their young—this image was used to indicate it was time for couples to marry. The Mei's chief officer acted as a Protector Lord (of the place). When Gao Xin went out, the Dark Bird left an egg, which Jian from the Song tribe swallowed, thus giving birth to Xie. Later kings considered the Mei building to be auspicious and so established sacrifices there. Changing the written form of the word *mei* from 媒 to 禖 (exchange of the original "female" semantic to that of "spirit tablet") represented its divinization.[42]

The deity (and prehistoric sage-king) Gao Xin 高辛 appears in Han texts also as Di Ku 帝嚳, one of the five divinities, identified during the Han period as descendant from the mythical original emperor of the Chinese people, Huangdi 黃帝 (Yellow Emperor). Gao Xin was associated in the Han ideology of Wuxing (the Five Agents: Wood, Fire, Metal, Water, Earth) with governing the cosmic Fire energy (which is assigned to the Chu ancestor Zhu Rong 祝融 elsewhere). Zheng Xuan's connection of the Gaomei and Dark Bird myths derived from the "Dark Bird" (*xuanniao* 玄鳥) ode preserved in the *Book of Odes*. In this ode, the Dark Bird was an emissary of the sky spirit Tian. The bird descended (*jiang* 降) to give birth to the Shang (people). Di, then, caused the founder ancestor of the Shang, Cheng Tang 成湯, to begin to set up a new state (after the destruction of the old state, the Xia 夏). While this ode does not mention the mother's name, it appears as Song 娀 in another ode with Di specified as the father.[43] In the *Chuci* and later versions of the myth, she is called Jiandi 簡狄. The *Shiji* goes further, not only explaining that the mother was from the Song 娀 people, but recounting that the bird dropped the egg by her when she was bathing with her sisters.[44] Granet understood these bathing rituals by groups of young women as "lustration nuptials," rituals of purification before marriage.[45] Zheng Xuan understood "Gaomei" to be both the god who supervised marriages and the place where sacrifices were proffered. He assumed from reference to the Dark Bird myth that such rituals must have begun in the distant past.

The association of a human sponsor or "chief officer" of the Mei site, a term later used for wedding matchmakers, helped to give the place historical legitimacy for Han scholars. However, most also understood Mei as the name of a spirit. Both the place and the god went by many names. The added appellation of "high" (*gao* 高) signified respect but perhaps also indicated a lofty open-air site with a lot of sunlight. Cai Yong 蔡邕 (132–192 CE) noted:

高, 尊也. 禖, 祀也, 吉事先見之象也. 蓋為人所以祈子孫之祀.
Gao is *zun* ("to be reverent") and *mei* is *si* ("to sacrifice"), representing that auspicious affairs are forthcoming. Perhaps this was a sacrifice for praying for descendants.[46]

Han scholar Lu Zhi 盧植 (d. 192) explained:

居明顯之處, 故謂之高. 因其求子, 故謂之禖. 以為古者有媒氏之官, 因以為神.
[Mei] is called *gao* because it was located in a brightly lit place and it is called *mei* because it is used to seek progeny. It is a divinity because there were Mei officers in antiquity.[47]

It is unclear whether these Han scholars had personal knowledge of such sites or were just drawing on popular legend or on texts now lost to us. Another name for the site and the god was "Jiao Mei" 郊禖, suggesting that there was an official Mei site in the "suburbs" (*jiao*) outside of a capital city.[48] Commentary by Mao Heng 毛亨 (second or third century BCE), known as the Mao commentary of the *Book of Odes*, notes on the ode "Birth of the People" that anciently Jiao Mei was established to get rid of childlessness and to seek a child. He then cited from the "Yueling" chapter of the *Ritual Records*:

去無子求有子, 古者必立郊禖焉. 玄鳥至之日, 以太牢祀于郊禖, 天子親往, 后妃率九嬪御, 乃禮天子所御, 帶以弓韣授以弓矢于郊禖之前.
On the day that the Dark Bird arrived and the large penned animal was sacrificed, the Son of Heaven personally "attended" to the concubines in the queen's retinue, who performed the ritual of mating with the Son of Heaven: carrying bow covers, they would be given sets of bow and arrows in front of Jiao Mei.[49]

The gift of a bow and arrows to a concubine whose bow case was "empty" symbolized her forthcoming pregnancy with a male child.

Kong Yingda 孔穎達 (574–648) suggests that local Mei sites were created to solve the problem that women needed to pray to relieve childlessness but at the same time were generally prohibited from leaving their homes (during his era, the late Sui–early Tang). Thus, he claims, the fertility ritual was combined with regular annual sacrifices (called *yinsi* 禋祀 the "pure sacrifice" mentioned in the classics)⁵⁰ and that when it came time to sacrifice, the Son of Heaven personally "escorted" the concubines so that those who weren't pregnant yet would become so.⁵¹ The Mao and Kong commentaries both emphasize the connection between Jiao Mei and reproduction and how the emperor's concubines who had not yet gotten pregnant regularly visited the shrine to pray for children. From Mao Heng's to Kong Yingda's era, the practice of rituals to relieve childlessness at Mei sites seems to have been active.

Scholars suggest that an old Zhou term, Bi Gong 閟宮 ("secluded building")—also the name of an ode—referred to a Gaomei–like place for the eastern state of Lu 魯. This ode, like the "Dark Bird" ode, describes the birth of the founder of a people. The first half (translated later) describes the building as well as details of the ritual and birth in a somewhat similar fashion to that in "Birth of the People." This song mentions her *de* (Tian-given power, virtue), a quality usually sought by men to prove their right to rule (through proper performance of military and sacrificial rituals). In the case of women, it may have been associated with their behavior within the clan. Texts as early as the Middle Western Zhou suggest that *de* was shared among the members of the same clan or people (*min de* 民德).⁵² Subsequent verses of this ode celebrate agricultural production, suggesting a link between female fertility and good harvests—also apparent in the Middle Western Zhou inscriptions:⁵³

> 閟宮有侐、實實枚枚.
> 赫赫姜嫄、其德不回.
> 上帝是依、無災無害.
> 彌月不遲、是生后稷、降之百福.
>
> The Secluded Building is silent, vast, and ornate,
> Majestic was Jiang Yuan, her *de* flawless,
> The High Lord was her support so there was no disaster, no harm.
> As the month drew near without delay, Hou Ji was born and there descended great good fortune.

The Mao commentary notes that the Bi Gong was "the shrine to Founder Ancestress Jiang Yuan," and he quoted an unknown Mr. Meng 孟氏 who claimed that Bi Gong was also known as a Mei Gong. Zheng Xuan later also understood the Bi Gong to be a shrine to Jiang Yuan:

周立廟自后稷為始祖，姜嫄無所妃（配），是以特立廟而祭之，謂之閟宮. 閟, 神之.

The Zhou set up a shrine to Hou Ji as the first ancestor; because (his mother) Jiang Yuan didn't have a mate, they set up a shrine to sacrifice just to her (instead of her husband as would be standard), calling it the Bi Gong, with *bi* signifying her divinization.⁵⁴

There were no specifics on what the shrine actually looked like but later scholars added further details. Qing scholar Ma Ruichen 馬瑞辰 (1777–1853) pointed out that the book *Lushi* 路史 (by Luo Mi 羅泌, twelfth century) linked the identity of the goddess Nüwa 女媧 (a popular Han goddess and creator of the cosmos with her male counterpart, Fuxi 伏羲) with the identity of a so-called Spirit Mei (Shen Mei 神媒). Ma also noted that in the *Fengsu tongyi* 風俗通義 it says that once Nüwa became a goddess called Nü Mei 女媒, she had the power to negotiate marriages. Then Ma went on to explain how despite the fact that the Bi Gong shrine was to Jiang Yuan, it became conflated with the Mei Gong shrine to Shen Mei. Basically, Jiang Yuan had to perform the traditional Jiao Mei role since, like all women (in Ma's time), she couldn't randomly leave her home. The name Mei Gong, he claims, comes from that legend.⁵⁵

Another Qing scholar, Chen Huan 陳奐 (1786–1863), also believed that Mei Gong was an ancient term, going back to the prehistorical era of the god-king Gao Xin (presumed father of the mother of the Shang progenitor). First, he notes that the Han dictionary, the *Shuowen*, defined the word *mei* 禖 as "to sacrifice" (*ji ye* 祭也), and then he explained the nature of the sacrifice, citing from the *Wujing yiyi* 五經異義, a selection of commentaries on the classics, presumably collected by the author of the *Shuowen* (but lost before being reconstructed from fragments by Qing scholar Chen Shouqi 陳壽棋, 1771–1834).⁵⁶ The *mei* sacrifice, he explained, was incorporated into the seven annual sacrifices that the kings made to Tian. It took place in mid-spring and involved the queen and concubines performing the Jiao Mei ritual at the Mei Gong.⁵⁷ Clearly, he was influenced by earlier commentaries on the "Bi gong" and the "Yueling." How ancient the rite really is, whether the Bi Gong was in fact a shrine for Jiang Yuan, and whether it was for a Mei rite, we will never know.⁵⁸ From the content of the "Bi gong" ode, however, we can confirm that the Bi Gong, like the Mei Gong, was associated with fertility and birthing and possibly located outside of cities. The worship of Jiang Yuan was similar to the worship of the legendary mother of King Wen, who like Jiang Yuan, gave birth to a progenitor.

The Mei rites may have involved unscripted "wild" meetings between boys and girls to increase the probability of having heirs. Late Warring States and Han texts record incidents of unfettered congress between boys and girls during spring festivals outside of the cities. These accounts were explored by scholars, such as Marcel Granet in the 1920s, before the advent of modern archaeology and the discovery of many new texts, such as the *Zigao*.[59] Even so, a review of some of the traditional sources does suggest a spring festival in which boys and girls met to improve the chances for female fertility. For example, a section discussing the role of the official titled the "Intermediary" ("Mei Shi" 媒氏) in the *Zhouli* 周禮 (a text finalized during the Han that described the ideal government) explains that:

> 中春之月，令會男女，于是時也，奔者不禁。. . . 司男女之無夫家者而會之.
> Mid-spring is the season when the boys and girls are called to meet together and those who run off together are not punished. . . . it was the responsibility of the Intermediary to bring together those without mates.[60]

In the "Ru guo" 入國 chapter of *Guanzi* 管子 (also consolidated during the Han):

> 凡國都皆有掌媒. 丈夫無妻曰鰥，婦人無夫曰寡; 取鰥寡而合和之，. . . . 此之謂合獨.
> All states have someone who handles *mei*. A man without a wife was called *guan* and a wife without a husband was called *gua*. To get the *guans* and the *guas* to join together harmoniously. . . . This is called "joining together the singles."[61]

Gao You 高誘 of the Eastern Han period quoted this text as an authority when he tried to explain the mention of Gaomei in the mid-spring section of the Warring States text *Lüshi chunqiu* 呂氏春秋.[62] Fertility rites involving a time of lovers' trysts clearly transgressed the standard mores of the Han when women were increasingly kept at home, separate from any mixing with the opposite sex except with one's father, brothers, or husband according to a strict Confucian social code. Yet the release from such strictures for the sake of social reproduction persisted in ancient records. It may also have drawn on ancient rituals that used such combined male and female iconography such as we saw in Fu Hao's tomb.

According the "Minggui" 明鬼 chapter of the text of fifth-century BCE thinker Mozi 墨子 (reconstructed from fragments preserved in later texts at various times in history), there were various festivals at different sites that incorporated the custom:

> 燕之有祖，當齊之社稷，宋之有桑林，楚之有雲夢也，此男女之所屬而觀也.
> The Zu festival of Yan, the She festival of Qi, the Sanglin festival of Song, and the Yunmeng festival of Chu, were where boys and girls met and enjoyed each other.[63]

According to scholars Guo Moruo 郭沫若 and Wen Yiduo, it was the same spirit (goddess) in charge of all the sites (called Gao Tang, Gaomei, and so forth).[64] The place-names with "Gao" in the title initially suggesting a type of site evolved into a general name for such festivals and finally into the names of the divinities or goddesses worshipped. It seems that early fertility rites that took place out in the wilds eventually evolved into more formal suburban sacrifices involving married women.

If we, based on our understanding of Jiang Yuan's ritual so far, take the place Chuanjiu in the *Zigao* bamboo text as a possible Gaomei site, then we can use details only preserved in the *Zigao* record to reconstruct the Warring States–period idea of the ancient rite. One detail is particularly revealing. Once she reached the site, instead of sacrificing large, specially bred animals as in the formal suburban sacrifice, she simply presented a weed. Such simplicity could be construed to be a reflection of her sincerity, as per a passage in the *Zuozhuan* (Yin 3) (tales of the Spring and Autumn period compiled possibly as early as the third or fourth century BCE), which provides other examples of purposely simple offerings.[65] However, research on the exact nature of the "weed" suggests that it was actually a specific plant chosen for its phallic shape, especially for use in Gaomei fertility rituals.

The weed was called *aohan* 芺攼 in the *Zigao*. Ao seems to have been a hollow-stemmed thistle. The word *han* was phonetically similar to words written 扞 or 捍 meaning "to protect, ward off." As a noun, we might read it as *gan* 竿, referring to a cluster of sprouts (as in bamboo). According to the *Shuowen*, the sprouts of the Ao were eaten in the Jiangnan 江南 region to repress *qi* 氣 (rising *qi* in the body indicated an illness; *qi* was the cosmic vapor that was understood by the third century BCE to have engendered life and all visible things; there were Yang *qi* and Yin *qi*).[66] These sprouts were also described in other early etymological dictionaries as standing up straight and strong from the earth. So, besides the medicinal properties of the sprouts, the phallic image of their piercing straight up through the earth and their representation of a cluster of new life forms (a Yang manifestation) may also have contributed to their symbolic function as an antidote to childlessness. An ode in the *Book of Odes* called "bamboo sprouts" ("Zhu gan" 竹竿) is also suggestive. In it a young woman of Wei 衛 is traveling to Qi 齊 to get married. The ode opens with the image of "long and straight bamboo rods" (*titi zhugan* 籊籊竹竿) that are dangled presumably for fishing into the Qi 淇 River that she follows on her way. While the middle of the ode expresses her longing for home, the ode ends with coy smiles and the tinkling of jade pendants, a metaphor for the meeting of lovers (*qiaoxiao zhi cuo, peiyu zhi nuo* 巧笑之瑳、佩玉之儺). Wen Yiduo pointed out that fish also were metaphors for boys and girls mixing, and that the dangling of the fishing pole into the water represented the sexual act and its resulting fertility.[67]

Phallic imagery in the fertility rite is also evident in the classic version of Jiang Yuan's performance of the rite preserved in the ode "Birth of the People." According to the ode, she "enacted the pure sacrifice and the annual sacrifice in order to not be without children" (*ke yin ke si, yi fu wuzi* 克禋克祀、以弗無子).[68] Zheng Xuan (following up on the Mao interpretation) explains that these rituals were performed to Shangdi at Jiaomei and that the negative *fu* 弗 "not be (one who)" must be read as *fu* 祓 "to get rid of, exorcise," as in to get rid of Jiang Yuan's childlessness.[69] In any case, it is apparent that the place Chuanjiu in the *Zigao* must have been a Gaomei–like place. Jiang Yuan's offering of a phallic-shaped sprout to the fertility goddess, like the dipping of the fishing rod into the fish-filled river, would be symbolic of the sexual act.

Phallic imagery in ancient China is not unknown and may even be basic to the graph used for "ancestor" *zu* 祖. Stone and ceramic phalluses (called *shizu* 石祖 or *taozu* 陶祖) have been found near Xi'an and elsewhere in northern China.[70] The "Liyi zhi" 禮儀志 chapter of the *Sui shu* 隋書 (written by Wei Zheng 魏徵, 580–643) notes that:

梁太廟北門內道西有石,文如竹葉,小屋覆之。宋元嘉中修廟所得。陸澄以為孝武時郊祺之石。

There was a stone on the west side of the inner passageway of the Grand Shrine (built in) the Liang dynasty (502–557).

It had a pattern of bamboo leaves and a tiny room one could walk into. During the Yuanjia period of the Song dynasty (Liu-Song Emperor Wu, 420–422), the stone was found during repairs to the shrine. Lu Cheng (422–493) believed that it was the Jiaomei stone (used) during the Xiaowu period (Han emperor Xiaowu, r. 141–87 BCE).[71]

From this account, we know that in the period shortly after the Han dynasty, scholars believed that bamboo-patterned stones were used in Han Gaomei rituals and that their use may have continued at least into the Liang period.

A conceptual link between bamboo, sexual organs, fertility, and birth has been preserved among some non-Sinitic peoples living in the southwestern area of modern-day China. Traditional customs of the Yi 彝 peoples in Longlin 隆林, Napo 那坡, and Funing 富宁 living in the areas of Guangxi and Yunan provide a link between bamboo tubes and birthing. When a woman was about to give birth, her husband and brothers had to chop out a two-foot-long section of bamboo tube to store the afterbirth. It was then plugged with banana leaves and hung on a tree branch. The Yi people who live in Songziyuan 松子園 (Chengjiang 澄江, Yunnan) once worshipped a "Golden Bamboo" 金竹 spirit, calling it "Golden Bamboo Granddaddy" 金竹爺爺. Women who were not pregnant went to bamboo forests in the mountains and prayed to it for children, staying out all night in a nearby shrine.[72] While we cannot prove that such relatively modern practices have preserved aspects of older rituals from the more northern regions, the pervasive nature of such rituals allows us to understand that tales of Jiang Yuan's ritual may in fact have reflected actual practices. Hou Ji's mother's presentation of an emblem representing the male sexual organ to the goddess as part of a fertility ritual may have been an older version of the later ritual presentation of an "arrow" to the concubine. Both rituals aimed for the woman to become pregnant with a male heir.

Another detail of the Jiang Yuan tale reveals that the act of presenting the tube to the spirit caused Jiang Yuan to see a toe print (*nai jian ren wu* 乃見人武). The term for toe print, *wu* 武 written as 𢗳 (composed of elements representing a dagger and a foot), is found in early paleographic records such as oracle bones or bronze inscriptions, but is generally used as a sobriquet for a grand person (e.g., ancestor king) and then by association to "military." By the Warring States period, however, it also represented a "toe print," possibly a loan for *min* 敏, which could also mean "big toe." In the ode "Birth of the People," both words *wu* and *min* were used together, producing the alliterative combination *mrəʔ-mrəʔ*. The *Erya* 爾雅 etymological dictionary (ca. third century BCE), which defines many of the odd word usages in the *Book of Odes*, explains: "In [the expression] 'stepping on God's toeprint,' [the word] *wu* means "imprint" (*lü di wumin, wu, ji ye* 履帝武敏, 武, 迹也). From this and the two versions of the legend popular during the late Warring States period, we can understand that Jiang Yuan's fertility ritual included stepping into a human "toe print" no doubt someplace out in the wilds. This ritual combined with prayer helped her get pregnant with the progenitor of the Zhou people. The situation is highly suggestive of the fertility festivals associated with Gaomei shrines. By the Han period, the toe print was described as from a "giant" (*juren* 巨人) or from Tian. We see a mix of terms in the *Zigao* version of the tale, which describes the toe print as human, yet she prayed to a Di. In the *Ode*'s version, the Di was Shangdi. However, some suggest this must have be the footprint of her husband Gao Xin, who was also sometimes referred to as a Di.

If we look more closely at the opening lines of the ode "Birth of the People" from the standpoint of the *Zigao* version, we can uncover more details of the ritual:

> 厥初生民、時維姜嫄.
> 生民如何、克禋克祀、以弗無子、履帝武敏歆.
> 攸介攸止、載震載夙、載生載育、時維后稷.
> When first the People were born, it was of Jiang Yuan.
> How did she do it? By presenting the pure wine and annual sacrifices to counter infertility, and stepping onto Di's big toe print.
> It (the print itself or good fortune coming from Di in the form of pregnancy) kept growing large, and when it stopped, she felt movement, and when it became still, she gave birth, producing this who is Hou Ji.[73]

From the various versions of the Jiang Yuan tale, we know that the woman performing the fertility ritual first traveled outside the city. Then she presented symbolic offerings possibly at a Gaomei shrine, followed by stepping on a deity's toe print while going into the bushes. This resulted in a divine conception. Only the cases where a semi-divine prehistorical or historical figure was conceived have become the subjects of the early tales. We find an oblique reference to a similar ritual performed by Confucius's mother recorded at the beginning of the Kong lineage history in the *Shiji*. In order to conceive him, she met a man in the wilds and prayed at Ni Hillock 尼丘.⁷⁴ Neither the *Shiji* nor the *Ode*'s versions of Hou Ji's birth provide a specific site, so it seems that the *Zigao* version was not well known. Later commentaries attempted to clarify a location for the magical event. For example, the *Chunqiu yuanming bao* 春秋元命苞, by Song Jun 宋均 (d. 76) (but collected from fragments by Qing publisher Ma Guohan 馬國翰, 1794–1857), claims that Jiang Yuan traveled to Bi Gong or possibly to Fusang 扶桑 (a site mentioned in the *Chuci* and *Shanhaijing* associated with a magical mulberry tree and the sunrise) where she stepped on a giant toe print and then gave birth in the Bi Gong.⁷⁵ Song Jun attempts to separate the functions of the Bi Gong and Gaomei (or Jiao Mei), suggesting that the former site was for giving birth after successful fertility rites had been performed at the latter site.

Another detail from the *Zigao* version supports the idea of a Gaomei fertility ritual in the wilds. The phrase "be selected on her own" (in other words, without an intermediary or by parental introduction) suggests a custom whereby girls did not marry until they were pregnant. Ancient accounts and modern anthropological research provides us with some corroboration for this idea. Among the Mosou people in Yunan and southern Sichuan, for example, there used to be a rite in which a woman not yet with child would light incense and pray at a stone phallus (a *shizu* 石祖), then lift her skirts and sit on it awhile before meeting up with men that night.⁷⁶

Fertility aids included phallic-shaped weeds, stone phalluses, special quivers, and "tubes"; they also included signs from nature, such as the arrival of the Dark Birds. We also find evidence for the wearing of certain amulets or eating particular foods from wild areas as catalysts for fertility in the *Shanhaijing*. According to the chapter on southern mountains, "Nanshan jing" 南山經, on the Niuyang Mountain 杻阳之山:

有獸焉, 其狀如馬而白首, 其文如虎而赤尾, 其音如謠, 其名曰鹿蜀, 佩之宜子孫.
[It] has wild beasts there that look like horses with white heads and are patterned like tigers with red tails. They wail as if singing a folksong. They are called "Lu Shu" 鹿蜀. One can wear (a symbol of) one as a pendant to get progeny.⁷⁷

According to the chapter on western mountains, the "Xishan jing" 西山經, on Chongwu Mountain 崇吾之山:

有木焉, 員葉而白枻, 赤華而黑理, 其實如枳, 食之宜子孫.
There is a tree there with round leaves and white sepals and with red flowers that are black on the inside. The fruit is like a citrus and can be eaten for progeny.[78]

In the chapter on the central regional mountains, the "Zhongshan jing" 中山經, on Qingyao Mountain 青要:

南望墠渚, 禹父之所化, 是多僕纍、蒲盧. 䰠武羅司之, 其狀人面而豹文, 小腰而白齒, 而穿耳以鐻, 其鳴如鳴玉. 是山也, 宜女子. 畛水出焉, 而北流注于河. 其中有鳥焉, 名曰鴢, 其狀如鳧, 青身而朱目赤尾, 食之宜子.
If you look south toward Chanzhu where Yu's father transformed (into a dragon), there are many vines and rushes. It is overseen by a Wuluo sprite that has a human head and leopard markings and a tiny waist and white teeth. It wears earrings like drum sticks and when it chirps it sounds like stone chimes. This mountain is good for getting daughters. A stream comes out of it and flows northward into the Yellow River. There are birds there called "Yao" 鴢 that look like owls with greenish bodies, vermillion eyes, and red tails. Eating them is good for getting sons.[79]

Many mountains mentioned were occupied or visited by different Di, usually one of the Five Di associated with different colors or stars, or famous sage-kings called Di. These Di were often associated with different colors such as white and yellow, or with the mythological founder Di of prehistory. Wearing or eating items from these sites had the power to increase fertility. Although the *Shanhaijing* does not record any tales about famous mothers traveling there to perform rites, the connection between sacred sites and fertility is still evident. Curiously, by the late Warring States period, the ancient legend of a woman being impregnated by Shangdi took on a prankster form. In the *Day Book* chapter "Jie jiu" 詰咎, playful ghosts come for women and girls, claiming to be the children of Shangdi down for a stroll or to take a wife (strips 39–42, back 3).[80]

In the *Chu ju*, the conception of the two sets of twins occurred in wild areas, one in a mountainous area and the other in a river region. No marriage ceremony is mentioned for the parents. Perhaps we might understand this legendary mating scene to be similar to the Gaomei rituals described in this chapter.

3

Mothers and Embryos

The term "mother" (*mu* 母) represented a revered status in ancient Chinese religion. It was a woman who had been addressed as "wife" (*fu* 婦) when alive and had provided descendants. Most women addressed as *mu* in the ancient Zhou bronze inscriptions were already ancestral spirits. Reaching the status of ancestor spirit required status in life and a loyal set of wealthy descendants to provide the requisite sacrifices necessary for nurturing the dead. Powerful male ancestors were envisioned as being up in the sky next to Di. It is unclear where elite female spirits were believed to reside as in later times they seem to be associated with the earth. In any case, a "mother" was recognized in terms of the heir she produced, and one of her key duties was to prepare or supervise the sacrifices in her husband's ancestral shrine. Teaching new wives how to prepare the sacrifices was also the job of mothers-in-law. There were many different types of ancestor worship practices in early times, and it is likely mothers were only worshipped in some of these. From the *Chu ju* text, we know that Chu female ancestors were worshipped in terms of their connection to fathers and sons.

In some sacrifices, particularly those connected to the Zhou kings during the ninth century BCE, a time of ritual innovation, we find documented rituals for heirs being promoted into the official positions of their ancestors. These also helped to maintain historical social structures of power.[1] These rituals, like later capping rituals, propelled the heirs symbolically into the position of their elders. The capping rituals (or pinning rituals in the case of women) also marked the time when they must marry, hence, marking the beginning of their socially reproductive roles. Although elite males were expected to participate in the military and the government as well as their lineage or family duties, the wives' prime duty was to produce heirs. From transmitted texts, we know that not all women who qualified as *mu* actually gave birth. They were also the "mothers" of the children of concubines, particularly boys.

In order to qualify for promotion into the position of one's elder, the heir had to accumulate enough social merit, *de* 德. This merit or inner power was awarded by the ancestral spirits to the heirs in exchange for sacrifices as well as for service to the ruler (who represented Tian or Heaven and was referred to as the Son of Heaven, *tianzi* 天子). By the time of the *Chu ju* text, aspiring men could earn *de* directly from Tian without requiring the intercession of the ancestral spirits. The high god associated with Tian called Di 帝 is associated by some scholars with the fourth-century BCE sky deity Taiyi 太一, sometimes translated as the Great Monad or Great Unity.[2] Because the title *di* was also applied to the spirits of the Shang kings, it is generally assumed that if Di or Taiyi had a gender it would have to be male.[3] However, a Chu text called *Taiyi Gives Birth to Water* (*Taiyi sheng shui* 太一生水), found in the upper middle Yangzi region of fourth-century BCE Chu, confuses the issue by referring to this high god as "mother" and linking "her" to water.[4] The fact that Taiyi was also associated with water, something that emerged from springs in the earth, reminds us of the early Shang semantic connections between graphs representing the words "to give birth, source, spring, special enclosure" discussed in chapter 1.

A key line regarding the nature of this mother figure in the Chu text records the belief that she "hides in water" before "moving according to the seasons" in an "all-encompassing" way, thus "becoming the beginning" and "the mother of all things."

> 是故太一藏於水, 行於時; 周而或(又)〔始[5], 以忌/已為〕萬物母.
> Thus, the Great Unity is stored in water and mobilized in the four seasons: cycling and beginning anew, it thereby acting as the mother of the myriad things.[6]

The greatest parallels to this representation of the mother god are found in the Daoist classic the *Daodejing* 道德經. Variations of this classic have been discovered in Chu and Han tombs, but with the sections focused on *de* and Dao reversed. These variations are referred to simply as the *Laozi* 老子, after the presumed great Daoist sage, who possibly lived around the time of Confucius at the end of the Spring and Autumn period, around the fifth century BCE. From the different versions of this ancient text, we learn that Dao, the Beginning, and Mother were parallel concepts. The *de* power, in contrast to the Dao, in most texts was associated with patrilineal social reproduction and, originally, with the power of Di (*tˤek, anciently a near homophone with *de*, *tˤək) and Tian (no phonetic similarity). By the Han period, there were five cosmic Di and there were five supernatural *de*, but we cannot prove that there was conceptual overlap due to the predominance in many spheres of the Han cosmic scheme of Wuxing (Five Agents). The male ancestors by the middle century of the Western Zhou period, at least by the ninth century BCE, were envisioned as members of Di's spirit bureaucracy. In later literature, *de* does not seem to be an inner power limited to men. But later the need to balance all Yang manifestations with Yin may have provided an impetus for creating matching female aspects of gods, including Taiyi.

The Daoist Mother by the fourth century BCE may already have represented in some circles a genderless creator, the abstraction of perfectly balanced Yin and Yang necessary to reproduce. From the Daoist classic we learn that she was the androgynous generator of everything: Heaven and Earth, All Under Heaven, All Things, including an aspect or "child" of herself, that is the Dao itself. The Mother was simply the symbolic point in time representing the split between existence and nonexistence, action and nonaction, form and formlessness, things and no-things, and other dualities.[7] In another Daoist text dating from around the same time as the *Chu ju*, called the "Eternal Prior" (*Hengxian* 恆先) and in the transmitted *Zhuangzi* 莊子, the cosmic beginning of all things was not referred to as "Mother" at all. The idea of "Mother" as the birth portal may have reflected an older or competing stratum of conceptual ideology at a time when all supernatural agencies were moving away from the domination by aristocratic lineages of ancestral spirits to a more abstract mechanized view of cosmic origin and change, what would become known as the Yin Yang Wuxing system. In this system the forces of Yin and Yang meshed with five primeval forces of Earth, Fire, Metal, Water, and Wood and the Five Directions of Center, South, West, North, and East (and later with visible planets). Before the Han time, there were only four "agents" (*xing*). Earth and Center (so important in the imperial era) did not yet exist.[8] A hint of the transition from a concrete metaphor for the Beginning, Mother, to an abstraction is evident in the vocabulary used in different Chu bamboo text versions of *Laozi*. In the transmitted versions, the Mother represents the embodiment of

Dao, the state of visible reality, the "having of things" (*you wu* 有物), but in the Guodian *Laozi* text A, strip 11, she is simply referred to as the state of "having form" (*you zhuang* 有狀).

This shift in wording is significant to our discussion of the role of the mother in ancient society. If we look at the uses of the word "form" (*zhuang*) in other late Warring States texts, the most interesting examples come from two different sections of the late Warring States text, the *Xunzi* 荀子, where we find it used in reference to a silkworm cocoon, the categories of "having of things," and to the dualistic phenomena of life and death:

> 有物於此，儳儳兮其狀，屢化如神，功被天下，為萬世文
> Here is a thing: How naked and bare its external form, [Y]et it continually undergoes spiritual transformation like a spirit. Its achievement covers the backs of the world.[9]

> 哀夫！敬夫！事死如事生，事亡如事存，狀乎無形影，然而成文
> How full of grief, how reverent this is! One serves the dead as one serves the living, those who have perished as those who survive, *just as though one were giving visible shape to what is without shape or shadow*, and so doing one perfects proper form.[10]

In the first example, the "form" of the silkworm, its cocoon specifically, is a member of the class of embodied things (*you wu*). The reference to providing covering and decor or "proper form" (*wen* 文) sets up the metaphor of creating the world to the female art of creating something out of nothing through textile weaving or birthing. There may have been a slight allusion to the female manufacture of all things in the *Taiyi sheng shui* text where the Mother "weaves" all things out of what is alternately empty and full.[11] The *Xunzi* passage goes on to refer to the usefulness of silk in completing proper ritual. This is somewhat related to the next passage in the sense that the writer, Xunzi (BCE 310–211?), was exclaiming how the perfectly performed ritual provided "form" for the dualist phenomena of life and death, surviving or not, the states of form and formlessness.

One curious note regarding the use of "form" (*zhuang* 狀 *dzaŋ-s*) is the fact that the ancient word was a near homophone with the ancient word used in the *Taiyi sheng shui* for "hide, conceal, store up" (*zang* 藏 *dzˤaŋ-s*). If we understand that ancient bamboo texts were most likely read out loud, it is possible that what the acolytes actually heard was that the Mother was "formed" in water, a primal substance, chaotic yet capable of stillness and movement.[12] It would fit with the theory of Yin in the Yin and Yang dualism of wet and dry, and, later, female and male.[13] Another way of understanding Taiyi might be as the form that encloses the Dao and ultimately gives birth to Water, which through a recursive cycling process produces the dualities Heaven and Earth, Yin and Yang, the Four Seasons, and so forth.[14] In this sense, the role of Mother as the "cocoon" out of which naked caterpillars (wrinkled like newborn babies) might emerge also symbolized the shaper of all things. This abstract sense remotely reflects the ancient image of babies, water, and sacrificial animals emerging from enclosure.

Embryonic Transformation

The earliest account of the formation of an embryo is found in a newly discovered bamboo text from the same cluster of fourth-century texts as the *Chu ju*. This book, called Tsinghua *Tang at Chi Gate* (*Tang zai Chimen* 湯在啻門), is one of a series of tales about the Shang founder king Cheng Tang consulting with the diviner/shaman/minister Yi Yin 伊尹 about questions of governance and philosophy.[15] In this text, Cheng Tang asks him about what "completes" (*cheng* 成) a person (*ren*), a state (*bang* 邦), earth (*di*), and sky (*tian*), in that order. In Warring States Ru 儒 (early Confucian) ideology, "completing" oneself involved self-cultivation ("techniques of the heart," *xinshu* 心術) through the practice of ritual music and other arts associated with "study" (*xue* 學).[16] Generally, this was understood as a process that involved nine stages, nine representing the peak Yang force in divination and the "completion" of a musical performance. This involved nurturing the *de* from inside oneself, shaping the inner "intention" (*zhi* 志) one was born with to become a fully formed ethical adult, a *chengren*. Since the goal is to become enlightened or "bright" (*ming* 明) enough to rule, or at least assist a ruler, the practitioner is assumed to be male. The Cai bronze inscription translated on pp. 27–28 suggests a female version of the practice, but the focus of "completing" a person was clearly on the potential heir, a male.

In the text *Tang at Chi Gate* (which many read as *Tang at Di's Gate*, since *chi* was an alternative way to write *di*, "god"), Tang is focused on how to prepare himself to take over from the failing Xia dynasty and create a new state, the Shang dynasty. The discussion of the elements that come together to form the embryo and then the stages of embryonic growth must be understood then as metaphors for internal transformation. In this sense, it is startlingly like the early medieval Daoist male practice of rebirthing the transcendent self in the form of the "ruddy infant" (*chizi* 赤子).[17] In this practice, the idea is to reverse the negative effect of actually having been physically born from a female human. It involves visualizing inside the body spiritual parents: an internal "dark" mother (called the "Dark Radiance Jade Maiden," Xuanguang yunü 玄光玉女), representing primordial Yin *qi* and equivalent to the Grandmother of the West (Xi Wangmu 西王母),[18] and a father, perhaps the Grandfather of the East (Dong Wangfu 東王父) or other celestial beings who represented pure Yang *qi*.[19] With the aid of nine key spirits (riding on top of a divine tortoise)[20] visualized between the two kidneys, after you enter the "Palace of the Great Abyss," you must envision "Taiyi of the Purple Palace, the Dark Maiden, and the Ruddy Infant."[21] Although it is the Jade Maiden of Mystic Radiance who is the mother of primordial *qi* of the Dao (Xuanguang yunü *zhe, dao yuanqi zhi mu ye* 玄光玉女者, 道元氣之母也),[22] the mother of the embryo is in fact the Daoist male practitioner himself.

The Tsinghua text describes the formation of the embryo as a process of harmonizing the *qi* of Five Flavors (*wu wei zhi qi* 五味之氣) to "complete a person" but also requiring the inner force of *de* to make him "radiant" (*guang* 光). Unfortunately, the text does not name what it means by the Five Flavors. Although the Five Flavors are referred to in other Warring States texts, they are not specified until Han times (as part of Wuxing theory), as sour, salty, spicy, bitter, and sweet (*suan, xian, xin, ku, gan* 酸咸辛苦甘). In the "Shuidi" 水地 chapter of the *Guanzi*, the Five Flavors are connected to the formation of the organs:

人, 水也. 男女精氣合, 而水流形. 三月如咀, 咀者何? 曰五味. 五味者何? 曰五藏. 酸主脾, 鹹主肺, 辛主腎, 苦主肝, 甘主心. 五藏已具, 而後生肉. 脾生隔, 肺生骨, 腎生腦, 肝生革, 心生肉. 五肉已具, 而後發為九竅: 脾發為鼻, 肝發為目, 腎發為耳, 肺發為竅, 五月而成, 十月而生.

People are water. When essential *qi* of males and females are joined together, the water flows and creates shape. In the third month, it is like paste. What is this paste? It is called the Five Flavors. What is this Five Flavors? It is called the Five Viscera: sour is the basis of the spleen, salty of the lungs, spicy the kidneys, bitter the liver, sweet the heart. Once the

Five Viscera are established, then fleshy parts grow. The spleen generates the separations, the lungs generate the bones, the kidneys generate the brain, the liver the skin, and the heart the muscle. Once the five fleshy parts are established, the nine cavities are created. From the spleen comes the nose, the liver the eyes, the kidneys the ears, and the lungs the openings. This process is completed in five months and then (the person) is born in the tenth month.²³

The Tsinghua text describes the Five Flavor generation process as beginning with the Jade Seed (*yuzhong* 玉種), which scholars agree must refer to semen:

唯彼五味之氣, 是哉以爲人, 其末(本?) 氣是謂玉種. 一月始(胎?) 蕩(揚?), 二月乃裏, 三月乃形, 四月乃骨(固?), 五月或(有?)收, 六月生肉, 七月乃肌, 八月乃正, 九月顯章(彰?), 十月乃成, 民乃時生. It's the *qi* of the Five Flavors that is what first makes up people, with the basic *qi* being called the Jade Seed. In the first month, it (the fetus) begins to beat (come alive); in the second month, then it forms the amniotic sac; in the third month, it forms a shape;²⁴ in the fourth month the bones²⁵ are formed (it solidifies?); in the fifth month, it receives (the influence of the Five Flavors?); in the sixth month, it fleshes out; in the seventh month, it develops skin; in the eighth month, it obtains the correct form (gender differentiation?);²⁶ in the ninth month, it becomes fully manifest; in the tenth month then it is complete, and that is when people are born.²⁷

Gil Raz, in a study of Han and medieval embryologies, has produced a useful chart comparing the stages of the embryo for each month.²⁸ He lists the stages mentioned in (1) the *Book of the Generation of the Fetus* (*Taichan shu* 胎產書) from the Mawangdui 馬王堆 tomb of 168 BCE discovered in Changsha, Hunan, and in studies by Donald Harper;²⁹ (2) the *Huainanzi* 淮南子 (written about thirty years later than the Mawangdui burial);³⁰ (3) the section on the fetus from the *Chanjing* 產經 (preserved in the Japanese collection *Ishinpō* 醫心方 dated to 982); and (4) the section on pregnancy from the *Huaishen* 懷身 (in the same collection). To these comparisons, we can add a selection from the *Wenzi* 文子 (an early Han Daoist text).³¹

The first and second months: In the Tsinghua text, the fetus is just begun in the first month, and it begins to have an amniotic sac (a "wrapping"). This is similar to "first formation" (*shi xing* 始形) in the *Huaishen* and to the "flowing and formation" in the *Taichan shu* and in the *Guanzi* selection translated earlier (for the first and second months). The fetus in the first month in the *Huainanzi* and *Wenzi* (but the second month in the *Taichan shu* and *Huaishen*) is described as "lard" (*gao* 膏) (in *Huaishen* the second month is "first lard," *shigao*). Perhaps this is similar to what is meant by "paste" (*ju* 咀) in the *Guanzi* passage. The *Chanjing* assigns "embryonic sac" (*peibao* 胚胞) to the first month and the "fetus" (*tai* 胎) to the second. The placenta (*guo* 裹, see the *Shuowen* definition for *bao* 胞) in the Tsinghua text is assigned to the second month.

The third month: In the *Huainanzi*, this is the "fetus" stage, and in the *Huaishen*, this is the "first fetal stage" (*shi tai*). The *Taichan shu* describes the fetus at this stage as "suet" (*zhi* 脂), but the *Chanjing* attributes "blood vessels" (*xuemai* 血脈) to it. In the Tsinghua text, it is simply "forming" (*xing*). The *Wenzi* describes it as *pei* 胚 ("embryonic"), much like the first month stage in the *Chanjing* (and second month in the Tsinghua text).

The fourth month: The Tsinghua text and the *Chanjing* both attribute bone formation to this stage. The *Wenzi* simply says "fetus" (*tai*). The *Huainanzi* refers instead to "muscle" (*ji* 肌).[32] The influence of the Wuxing cycle asserts itself at this point on the *Taichan shu* and the *Huaishen* accounts (except in both there are six not five elements, the sixth being "stone"). Both link the fourth month to Water (an element considered basic to humans in the *Guanzi*). Water is basic to "blood" (*xue* 血) in both texts.

The fifth month: This is the stage in the Tsinghua text that the fetus "receives" (*shou* 收) something, perhaps the influences of the Five Flavors that form its viscera (in the *Huaishen*, from the fourth through ninth months, the fetus "receives" (*shou* 受), the essence (*jing* 精) of the six different elements (Water, Fire, Metal, Earth, Wood, and Stone), each responsible for a different part of the body, but not of the viscera. It is possible then that this is more in line with what the fetus "received" in the Tsinghua text too as the viscera are never mentioned. The *Taichan shu* and the *Huaishen* link the element Fire and *qi* to the fifth month (it is perhaps significant that the archaic graph for *qi* included the "fire" semantic, suggesting that this is an association that can be traced back to the fourth century BCE). The *Wenzi* and the *Huainanzi* accounts both claim that tendons (*jin* 筋) are formed at this stage.[33] The *Chanjing* simply says "movement" (*dong* 動; this appears in the eight month in the *Huainanzi*).³⁴

The sixth month: The Tsinghua text simply refers to "generating flesh" (*sheng rou* 生肉). The *Wenzi* and *Huainanzi* both have "bone" for this stage, and the *Taichan shu* and *Huaishen* have the element Metal and "tendons" (*jin*). The *Chanjing* merely notes that the "form is complete" (*xing cheng*), which is reminiscent of the *Guanzi* assertion for the fifth month.

The seventh month: The Tsinghua text puts "muscles" (*ji* 肌) at this stage (note the *Huainanzi* placed this in the fourth month). The *Huainanzi* now claims that the fetus is basically "complete" (*cheng*); the *Wenzi* has the "form is complete" (*xing cheng*; note the *Chanjing* said this for the sixth month). The *Chanjing* claims that "hair" (*maofa* 毛髮) develops at this stage.³⁵ The *Taichan shu* and *Huaishen* attribute the element Wood to the development of bones.

The eight month: The Tsinghua text has "correct form" (*zheng* 正), a concept not repeated in any of the other texts. The *Huainanzi* and the *Wenzi* both simply say "movement" (*dong*), and the *Taichan shu* and *Huaishen* attribute Earth to the development of skin (*fuge* 膚革). The *Chanjing* notes the formation of "light in the pupils" (*tongzi ming* 瞳子明).³⁶

The ninth month: The Tsinghua text refers to the quality of "showing, manifest" (*xianzhang* 顯彰), perhaps like the light in the pupils representative of human consciousness. The *Taichan shu* and the *Huaishen* attribute the element Stone to the development of hair at this stage. The *Huainanzi*, *Wenzi*, and *Chanjing* all remark on the "quickening" (*zao* 躁) or "beating into the stomach" (*gu ru wei* 鼓入胃), which perhaps refers to either the intensified movement of the fetus or the stronger contractions of the uterus. Then by the tenth (lunar) month, the child is born.

We can see from these comparative accounts that similar fetal attributes were often claimed to develop at different stages. In some ways, the numerology of the counting of the months seems to be more important than exactly which attribute appears at which month. Despite the irregular specifics, it would seem that the accounts, moving from descriptions of lumps of lard to the appearance of hair, must be based on observation, possibly from miscarriages or cases of cutting open the pregnant belly. We discuss the possibility of ancient attempts to perform cesareans in chapter 6.

4

Controlling the Pregnant Body

Once diviners determined that a woman was in fact with child, it was critical to the household to monitor the outcome of the pregnancy. Numerous environmental and supernatural factors could influence the pregnant body in ancient China and the type of child it bore. Some of the oldest influential spirits, besides ancestors, where those of time itself.

Time and Divination

Ritual time was regulated by a sixty-day cyclical calendar. This consisted of an interlocking rotation of two sets of signs: one consisting of ten "sun" or day signs (*ri* 日), later known as "Heavenly Stems" (*tiangan* 天干), and twelve astral signs (*chen* 辰), later known as "Earthly Branches" (*dizhi* 地支). Units of time had spiritual agency, and even as far back as the Shang period, diviners predicted auspicious or inauspicious outcomes according to the signs of certain days. In the Shang and early Zhou periods, the posthumous names of powerful ancestral spirits, both male and female, were assigned day signs. These signaled the days they would receive sacrifices and may have also been the days they could most influence the bodies of their descendants. Although the Shang bone inscriptions are cryptic, we do see appeals to particular female ancestors regarding the outcome of a birth, not only whether the birth will be successful but whether the gender would be male. In each case, the clients of the diviners were royal women. The focus on political reproduction in these records is obvious; a few of the records show direct involvement of the king.

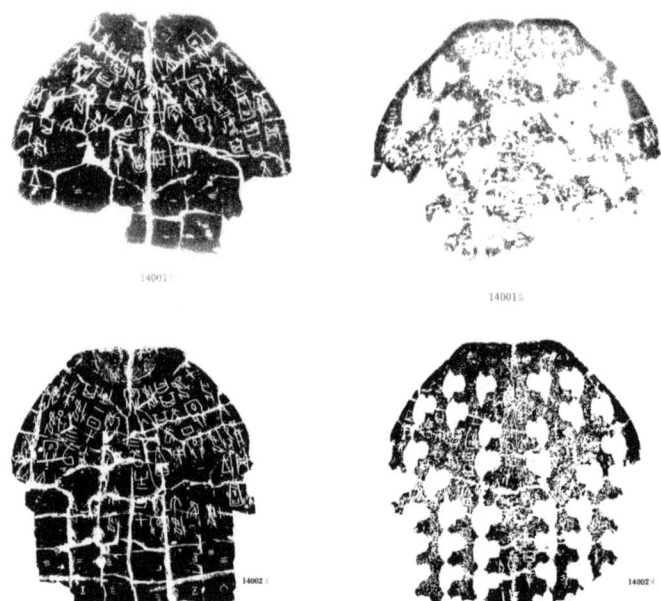

Figure 11. Oracle bones with birth divination from *Heji* 14001 and 14002 recto and verso of each tortoise plastron. The back sides show the holes drilled into the bone to create mantic crack images with a hot poker. (Guo Moruo et al. 1978–1982, vol. 5, 1982–1983).

There are many oracle bone records concerning the birthing experiences of royal women, but none are as famous as those of Fu Hao, King Wu Ding's wife. In two famous examples on tortoise plastrons, numbered 14001 and 14002 in the *Heji* collection, we see diviners prognosticating on certain specified days. A smooth birth was considered "fortunate" (*jia* 嘉) (in other records a "smooth" birth is referred to as *yun* 允). The auspicious days for birthing sons seem to be Ding 丁 or Geng 庚 "sun" or "stem" signs (days 4 and 7). For girls, Jia and Bing days (1 and 2) do not seem to be auspicious (or perhaps the end of the lunar month is inauspicious?).

Heji 14001 (front side):

王寅卜，殼貞:婦[好]娩嘉; 王占曰: 其惟[X]申娩吉嘉; 其惟甲寅娩不吉; 罨惟女.
Crack-making on a Renyin day, Que prognosticated: "Fu [Hao's] birthing will be fortunate." The king interpreted:

"Perhaps the birth will be on a [X graph unclear]-shen day and be auspicious and fortunate; perhaps the birth will be on a Jiayin day and be inauspicious; it follows[1] that it was a girl.

壬寅卜, 瀫貞: 婦好娩不其嘉; 王占曰: 孔不嘉其嘉不吉于 . . . 若茲廼葬.
Crack-making on a Renyin day, Que prognosticated: "Fu Hao's birthing will perhaps be unfortunate?" The king interpreted: "In the case of it being unfortunate, or perhaps being fortunate but not auspicious, in . . . such a case then she will be buried."

Heji 14002 (front side):

甲申卜, 瀫貞: 婦好娩嘉; 王占曰: 其惟丁娩嘉; 其惟庚娩弘吉; 三旬又一日甲寅娩不嘉惟女
Crack-making on a Jiashen day, Que prognosticated: "Fu Hao's birthing will be fortunate." The king interpreted: "Perhaps the birth will be on a Ding day and the birth will be fortunate, or perhaps it will be on a Geng day and the birth will be greatly auspicious." On the thirty-first day, a Jiayin day, she gave birth. It was not fortunate. It was a girl.

甲申卜, 瀫貞: 婦好娩不其嘉; 三旬又一日甲寅娩身不嘉隹女.
Crack-making on a Jiashen day, Que prognosticated: "Fu Hao's birthing will perhaps be unfortunate." On the thirty-first day, Jia day, she gave birth. It was not fortunate. It was a girl.

Heji 14002 (reverse side):

王占曰: 其惟丁娩嘉; 其庚[X]吉.
The king interpreted: "The birth will perhaps be fortunate and on a Ding day, or perhaps [X unclear] be auspicious on a Geng day."

Scholars have assumed from these records that all births of girls were considered unfortunate.[2] Although no doubt potential heirs were most valued, the situation may have involved a finer calculation of balancing the right days with the gender of the child. For example, Fu Hao, who seemed to give birth to many children, gives birth to a girl on a Guisi 癸巳 day and a son on a Gengzi 庚子 day without further comment.[3]

The term "unfortunate" might also have referred to the difficulty of the birth instead of just the gender of the child.

Some female ancestor spirits were called upon as aids, but in the case of difficult experiences, they were thought to have cursed the woman. In the case of curses, shamans (*wu* 巫) were then required to perform exorcisms or purification rituals for the protection of the birthing mother and the child. A cursed birth could result in death.[4] Jia days seem to have been particularly dangerous. On *Heji* 13996 after the diviner Bin cracked the bone on day Dingyou regarding whether Fu Hao's birthing would be fortunate, the king interpreted: "Perhaps it will be a Jia day birth and there will be a curse and . . . 其惟甲娩有祟有[X]."

By the fourth and third centuries BCE, with the rise of the Yin (weak, dark) and Yang (strong, light) system of binomial *qi* forces (which replaced the earlier system of ancestral forces), the days marked with astral signs ("branches") also became gendered. Male days were also called "hard" (*gang* 剛), or "male (animal)" (*mu* 牡) days and included *zi* 子, *yin* 寅, *mao* 卯, *si* 巳, *you* 酉, and *xu* 戌 (day numbers: 1, 3, 4, 6, 10, 11). Female days were also called "weak" (*rou* 柔) and "mare" (*pin* 牝) and included *chou* 丑, *chen* 辰, *wu* 午, *wei* 未, *shen* 申, *hai* 亥 (day numbers: 2, 5, 7, 8, 9, 12).[5]

The gender of the days influenced the outcome of burials, marriages, earthworks, and illness. Days in turn were divided into finer slices of male and female influence, times of day or night, phases of the moon, months, seasons, and so forth—aspects of male- and female-influenced time were also reflected in the earlier fourth-century BCE stalk divination bamboo manuscript called the *Shifa* 筮法. The Fangmatan *Day Book* notes that most tricky times are when the sun is rising and falling and generally at night. The male *qi* is strongest at dawn and the female at midnight.[6] Different Hai 亥 days during the spring, autumn, or winter are good for burying women (but others will harm living women if the earth is disturbed). Months were divided into male and female as well. It was most auspicious for a male to bring in a wife on a "male day" in a "female month," but it was best for a woman to marry on a "female day" of a "male month." The system generally corresponded to Yin and Yang days, hard and soft days, and odd and even months mentioned in transmitted texts.[7] The system of sixty ritual calendar days (binomial signs of "stem" + "branch") were further divided into "upper" and regular Yang and Yin days and divided by the Five Agents (*wuxing*)—with Metal, Water, and Wood Hai 亥 days leading the rotation. In some Qin almanacs, these are also matched with five musical modes, numbers, and time, all factors in the larger calculation of fate.[8]

The fates of children born on particular days of the calendar are listed and range from determinations of future afflictions, length of life, career, temperament, physical beauty, wealth, whether they will be motherless or orphaned, and so forth. In the almanacs, concern over birthing outcomes is paramount: of six influential days, with special names such as "Bind" (*jie* 結), Yang, "Crossover" (*jiao* 交), "Harm" (*hai* 害), Yin, and "Establish" (*jian* 建), the first and last are alternatively inauspicious for boys or girls, and one, the Yin day, is auspicious for marriage. The "Binding" day is inauspicious for the completion of any project, much less the production of more than one son. Of six extended days, with various names such as the Outer Yang, Outer Harm, Outer Yin, "Beat" (*Ji* 擊), "Sharp Radiance" (*Guai guang* 夬光), and "Elegant" (*Xiu* 秀) days, two of them, Beat and Sharp Radiance, resulted in across-the-board bad (Beat) or good (Sharp Radiance) fates for infants. One, the Elegant day, is inauspicious for younger brothers specifically, even if all other signs suggest an auspicious birth.[9] In another list it claims that a child born on an Elegant day will become an immortal, but a child born on a Yin day will become a robber.

Other lists of days calculate the inauspicious and auspicious nature of issues concerning a relatively wealthy household, one with slaves, goods to bring to market, buildings, and farming enterprises. In this context, marrying a wife was auspicious on a Ping 平 day, which was generally a good day for starting new projects and bringing new people into the family. But elsewhere a Jiao 敫 day or a "Perilous Yang" (*weiyang* 危陽) day had the complete opposite effect. The birth of babies was included in the category of new people added to the family. Some days, such as "Discard" (*che* 徹) day, were safe for marriage, but any infants born on these days would die, suggesting that while both bringing in a wife and birthing a baby resulted in adding new people to the family, they were not equal in auspiciousness on certain days.[10] The assumption may have been that the infant should be male and therefore the relative male and female value of the day would influence the new people in different ways.

Slices of the day were also potent in terms of producing a male or female baby. For example, in the third-century BCE *Day Book* from Fangmatan, sixteen sections of the day alternated the possibilities of producing a male or female:[11]

> The time when the sun just reached the horizon (*pingdan* 平旦) produced a female, but at actual sunrise (*richu* 日出) a male; at breakfast time (*sushi* 夙食) a female, but at dinner time (*moshi* 莫食) a male; at noon (*rizhong* 日中) a female, but

just past noon (*ri guozhong* 日過中) a male; in the afternoon (*ri ze* 日則) a female, but deeper into the afternoon (*ri xiabie* 日下別) a male; just before sunset (*ri wei ru* 日未入) a female, but a sunset (*ri ru* 日入) a male; at dusk (*hun* 昏) a female, but at night (*yemo* 夜莫) a male; just before midnight (*ye weizhong* 夜未中) a female, but at midnight (*yezhong* 夜中) a male; and, after midnight (*ye guozhong* 夜過中) a female, but when the cock crows (*ji ming* 雞鳴) a male.

Other aspects of time were influential. During the Western Zhou period (1046–771 BCE) auspiciousness was calculated by the phase of the moon as well as the cyclical segenary day sign. The most auspicious time for casting a bronze was on day Dinghai 丁亥 (number 24 out of the sixty) during the days when the moon was reappearing early in the lunar month, called "Early Auspicious" (*chu ji* 初吉). The auspicious nature of this lunar cycle is replicated in the fourth-century BCE *Shifa*, where we see a cosmic pairing of husband and wife spiritual agencies during the month to give birth to the new lunar moon.

This *Shifa* manuscript employs the interrelationships between sets of male and female trigrams that appear in divination. Basically, a trigram is a reflection of Yin and Yang binomial energies reflected in later times by three broken or unbroken lines familiar as the basic components of the sixty-four hexagrams that appear in transmitted versions of the *Book of Changes* (the *Zhouyi* 周易 or *Yijing* 易經). Prior to the Han period, trigrams and hexagrams (both called *gua* 卦) were written as number series. A trigram was female if one out of the three lines was an even number and male if it was an odd number. The exceptions were the most powerful male and female trigrams, which were all odd or all even numbers.[12] The actors in the tale of the birth of the moon include (using the more traditional *gua* representations): Qian ☰, Kun ☷, Xun ☴, and Gen ☶. In a Han text attached to the *Zhouyi*, called *Explications of the Gua* (*Shuogua* 說卦), these trigrams are assigned hierarchical statuses equivalent to Husband, Wife, Eldest Girl, Youngest Boy.[13]

In section 22 (strips 39–40), the text explains:

凡乾, 月夕吉. 坤, 月朝吉. 坤, 晦之日逆乾以長巽; 入月五日舍巽, 乾坤長艮; 旬, 乾坤乃各返其所.

In all cases, Qian is auspicious at the end of the month and Kun is auspicious at the beginning of the month. On the day of the new moon Kun invites Qian to linger at Xun. As the moon enters its fifth day, they quit Xun. Qian and Kun linger at Gen. On the tenth day, Qian and Kun then each return to their (original) places.

Qian 乾, a trigram consisting of 111, represents the husband, and Kun (666) is his wife. At the end of the month, when there is no apparent moon, the wife invites the husband to linger in the position of Xun, a powerful female force that was also associated with spring and the auspicious direction of southeast. Once the moon begins to brighten again, they move to Gen, the youngest boy trigram, and finally by mid-month are back in their original places.

We see some of these same actors appear in a divination regarding determining the gender of a forthcoming child. In section 12 (strips 19–21) of the *Shifa*, we find a series of four trigrams represented by 666, 166, 116, 161, that is, the trigrams Kun 坤, Gen 艮, and Xun 巽. The number 161 represented the middle-ranked female, Li 離. Interestingly, however, the diviner creates a new trigram out of the six lines, 66[616]6, in the first line to determine the sex of the baby. The number 616 represents the middle-ranked male, Kan 坎 ☵:[14]

> 凡男, 上去二, 下去一, 中男乃男; 女乃女.
> In any case for a male, the (trigram) above must expel two (lines), and the (trigram) below expels one (line), so that (there is a) center (trigram), if (the central trigram) is male then (the baby) will be male, if (the central trigram) is female then (the baby) will be a female.

In the *Shifa*, the four seasons, the sun and astral signs (*ganzhi*), as well as the appearance of special numbers could all affect the auspicious nature of the trigram array. How the numbers were generated is a mystery. It is possible that the system was very ancient, going all the way back to the Shang period, as number series have been found on oracle bones as well as Western Zhou period pottery and bronze vessels. The last line of the *Shifa* reinforces the idea that proper divination was done with stalks.[15] However, dice have also been found in a third-century BCE tomb roughly in the same region the *Shifa* is believed to have come from.

The *Shifa* never includes the numbers 2 and 3 but does claim a special significance for the odd numbers of 5 and 9 and the even numbers of 4 and 8. It links these specially derived numbers to time and particular "line images" (*yaoxiang* 爻象) (section 29, strips 52–59). For even numbers 4 and 8 the images generally involve moisture or round containers, what we would expect for Yin *qi* (although the *Shifa* does not use Yang and Yin to describe either trigrams or numbers; nor does it refer to *qi*). The Yin *qi*-type numbers surround the Yang *qi*-type numbers. So, the metaphors for 8 and 4 surround those for 5 and 9. For some reason, 4 is listed last and 8 first, cocooning the odd numbers and Yang images:

> 八為風、為水、為言、為飛鳥、為腫脹、為魚、為罐筩。在上為醪，下為汰。
> (The line images) for 8 are wind, water, words, flying birds, swellings, fish, measuring cylinders; (when 8 appears) in the upper (trigram), it is alcohol (with sediment), and in the lower (trigram) it is wash water.[16]

> 四之象為地、為圓、為鼓、為珥、為環、為踵、為雪、為露,為霰。
> (The line images) for 4 are ground, circles, drums, earrings, circlets of jade, heels, snow, dew, hail.

Diviners had to consider these mantic images if these numbers appeared when he was calculating the numerical sequences for the trigrams.

The male and female dichotomy of cosmic influence is also apparent in the body diagram in section 24 of the *Shifa*. Different parts of the body are marked with the eight trigrams. Typical of a late Warring States conservative view of male "outer" and female "inner" social roles, the inner spaces of the body are all marked with female trigrams and the outer spaces with the male (notably this is in direct contrast to the aforementioned array of images linked to mantic numbers).

The body diagram from top to bottom (with gendered social roles added from the *Shuogua* text):

```
111  乾  Qian  ☰  (the top of the head)—husband
616  坎  Kan   ☵  (ears)—middle boy
166  艮  Gen   ☶  (lower arms and hands)—younger boy
611  震  Zhen  ☳  (below the knee and feet)—older boy
611  兌  Dui   ☱  (mouth)—younger girl
666  坤  Kun   ☷  (chest)—wife
161  離  Li    ☲  (abdomen)—middle girl
116  巽  Xun   ☴  (crotch)—older girl
```

This trigram marked body is set inside a circular array of trigrams that also correlate to time and space as explained by the surrounding text. South, the most auspicious direction is above the head and associated with Fire as one might expect from popular Han cosmologies (possibly due to the Chu or southern origin of the manuscript versus the northern origins of the *Zhouyi*). But, unlike Han correlations, the *Shifa* assigns a male trigram, Kan, to this direction, and not its opposite, the female Li. Li is placed below the body in the North and linked to Water. The figure's right side was to the East, dominated by male trigrams Zhen and Wood (with Xun to the southeast and Gen to the northeast), and its left side to the West, dominated by female trigram Dui and Metal (with Qian to the southwest and Kun to the northwest). Most of the female trigrams, such as Kun, Li, and Dui, were linked to darkness, wet, metal, except for Xun. Xun was associated with spring, southeast, and the site for conceiving the moon. It was also linked to the region of the body for birthing. In the following discussion of curses, we also see that Xun is linked to birthing twins, a concept relevant to our exploration of the mythologies behind the *Chu ju* account.

In a third-century BCE *Day Book* from Shuihudi 睡虎地 in Yunmeng 雲夢, Hubei, there appears a body diagram with a similarly splayed body but with no trigrams and no inner spaces delimited.[17] In fact there were two diagrams, one for winter and autumn and one for summer and spring, each with different parts of the outside marked with one of the twelve astral signs (*dizhi*). These determined the fate of the child born on particular days. Basically, the twelve signs are listed in order (1–12: Zi, Chou, Yin, Mao, Chen, Si, Wu, Wei, Shen, You, Xu, Hai) moving clockwise beginning with the right hand in the Yang months (Summer/Spring) and with the right foot in the Yin months (Winter/Autumn). If we assume the head is to the South and the body faces outward as in the *Shifa* diagram, we see the following correlations:

	Summer/Spring	**Winter/Autumn**
Top of the head:	Mao 卯 (male)	Si 巳 (male)
Right ear (neck):	Yin 寅 (male)	Chen 辰 (female)
Left ear (neck):	Chen 辰 (female)	Wu 午 (female)
Right shoulder:	Chou 丑 (female)	Mao 卯 (male)
Left shoulder:	Si 巳 (male)	Wei 未 (female)
Right hand:	Zi 子 (male)	Yin 寅 (male)
Left hand:	Shen 申 (female)	Wu 午 (female)
Right armpit:	Hai 亥 (female)	Chou 丑 (female)
Left armpit:	Wei 未 (female)	You 酉 (male)
Right foot:	Xu 戌 (male)	Zi 子 (male)
Left foot:	Shen 申 (female)	Xu 戌 (male)
Crotch:	You 酉 (male)	Hai 亥 (female)

The text explains:

> 人字：其日在首，富貴難勝殹，夾頸者貴．在奎者富．在掖（腋）者愛．在手者巧盜．在足下者賤．在外者奔亡．女子以巳字，不復字．
>
> As for the birth sign of a person, if the sign is the one on the head, then he will be a wealthy noble and difficult to overpower. If it is by the neck, he'll be rich. If it is by the armpit, he'll be loving. If it is at the hand, he'll be crafty and a bandit. If it is at the foot, he'll be a thief. If it is on the outside (the shoulder), then he'll run away. If a woman gives birth on a Si day, she will never give birth again.

The dire consequences for a woman who gives birth on a Si day (a male day, the fifth in the sequence of twelve) mentioned here do not match predictions for Si days elsewhere in the Shuihudi *Day Book*. Some babies born on Si days have happy futures. But Jisi 己巳 days are categorically bad:

> 凡己巳生，勿舉，不利父母，男子為人臣，女子為人妾．
>
> Do not raise any child born on a Jisi day. (Such children) will not benefit the parents: boys will become servants and girls will become concubines.[18]

The influence of ghosts on this day is also mentioned:

> 己巳生子，鬼，必為人臣妾．
>
> A child born on a Jisi day will be a ghost and must become a servant or a concubine to others.[19]

The influence of male and female days rotated according to season. Unlike with the trigrams, which have a clear numerical rationale (the appearance of odd or even numbers) for their male or female qualities, the gender assignments for the astral signs do not seem to be regular. The sequence does not follow the odd-and-even number pattern or even alternate rhythmically in any way: 1 Zi (M), 2 Chou (F), 3 Yin (M), 4 Mao (M), 5 Chen (F), 6 Si (M), 7 Wu (F), 8 Wei (F), 9 Shen (F), 10 You (M), 11 Xu (M), 12 Hai (F). The intrinsic male or female qualities of each sign must have some as yet unknown cultural associations, perhaps some of which were quite ancient.

In terms of the body diagram, we note that no matter whether during the Yin months of winter and autumn or the Yang months of summer and spring, the sign at the head is always male. Moving down the sides of the body, we find that both sides of the neck are female in the Yin seasons but only the left side in the Yang seasons. The shoulders are alternately dominated by male on the right during the Yin seasons and on the left during the Yang seasons (and vice versa for the female signs). The right hand is dominated by male signs no matter what season (and the left by the female). Both right and left armpits, on the other hand, are dominated by the female in all seasons, but the left armpit is dominated by a male sign during the Yin seasons (with a female sign in the right armpit during Yang seasons). Notably, the pelvic area (naturally associated with birth) was dominated by a female sign during the Yin seasons and a male sign during the Yang seasons. In the *Shifa* the pelvic area was influenced only by a female trigram, Xun 巽, the "eldest sister" of the trigram family (also associated with spring and the conception of the moon). Notably the two signs that appear in the crotch area in the Shuihudi diagram, *hai* and *you* were matched with female trigrams (Dui and Li) in in section 27 of the *Shifa*.[20] The power of female trigrams, particularly Xun, will be further discussed in the next section on curses.

Curses, Stars, and the Gendered Cosmos

Just as gods could provide fertility and auspicious births, capricious ghosts and spirits of all types (human, environmental, natural) could destroy them. Diviners had to determine the supernatural source of infertility, miscarriages, difficult labors, and deaths.[21] Oracle bone records attest to curses by Di, ancestors, legendary kings, mountains, rivers, directions/ regions (North, West, East, South), among others. These same categories of supernatural agency are apparent in fourth-century BCE divination accounts.[22] In Chu bamboo records, the most powerful and influential deities were the recently deceased ancestors. Anonymous ghosts were also greatly feared. Also influential were astral deities such as Taiyi or his Yin persona, the Occluded Tai (Shi Tai 蝕太)—understood as an early version of the Grand Yin (Tai Yin 太陰), linked in the Han time with the North, Water, and the Mother, and possibly as an invisible version of Taiyi (whose role as "mother" is expressed in the text *Taiyi Gives Birth to Water*).[23] Curses could also come from earth deities linked to altars in built and outside spaces.[24] Aspects of the residence, such as bedrooms, walkways, or gates, could be nefarious influences. Teams of diviners helped householders solve their problems. They employed multiple methods routinely each year or in cases of acute need to track down the sources of dysfunction and then to settle on the proper way to dismiss them, through sacrifices of food (particularly of specially raised animals), jade, or clothing, or different methods of exorcism upon the subject's body or residence.[25]

Trigrams could be diagrams for figuring out the sources of curses. In section 26 of the *Shifa*, sources of curses (*sui* 祟) are listed for each trigram. The sources, like the "images" of odd and even numbers, reflect Yin- and Yang-type natures. The list begins with the husband trigram, Qian, then goes to the wife trigram, Kun, and then goes by rank, alternating male and female but beginning with the youngest instead of the oldest. This pattern of listing the trigrams is seen elsewhere in the *Shifa*, supporting the idea of a reversal in motion caused by the strong female presence of Kun (666). We notice that in some sections of the *Shifa* concerning travel or military action, if the series of numbers moves from 1s to 6s (Yang to Yin) then the diviner advises the client to not proceed with his plan of action or to even return home; whereas if the numbers move from 6s to 1s (Yin to Yang) then the action can proceed forward. So, it seems that the currents of Yang and Yin influence are seen as the other's inverse in the fourth century BCE.

In the curses section, we also notice the effect of the unusual numbers of 4, 5, 8, 9. They pack an extra Yin and Yang diagnostic power to the trigram arrays. In the following, we will review the curses associated with the female trigrams and focus on the lines depicting curses associated with women, including those who died giving birth:[26]

> 坤祟: 門行, 純乃母, 八乃奴以死、乃西祭, 四乃縊者. [slip 44]
> The Kun curse: (the influence of) doorways and passageways; if (the stalk throw) produces all of one (type of Yin number for each line), then it is the mother; if (the throw) produces an 8 (for the Yin line), then it is a slave who died or from (the performance of) the sacrifice to the West; if (the throw) produces a 4, then it is one who died by strangulation.

> 兌祟: 女子大面端虩死, 長女為妾而死. [slip 46]
> The Dui curse: (the influence of) a girl who died of fright of a head with an over-large face;[27] the eldest girl who became a concubine and died.

離祟: 熱溺者, 四緫者, 一四一五長女殤, 二五夾四辜者. [slip 48]
The Li curse: (the influence of) people who were burned or drowned; (throwing a 4 (indicates) it is one who died by strangulation; (throwing) one 4 and one 5 indicates it was an elder girl who died early; (throwing) two 5s around a 4 (indicates) one who died by being quartered.

巽祟: 字殤, 五八乃巫, 九柆孿子, 四非狂、乃緫者. [slip 50]
The Xun curse: (the influence of) one who died early in childbirth; if (the throw) produces a 5 and an 8 then, it is a shaman; if a 9, then it is one (who died from) a split-side birth of twins;[28] if a 4, then it is one who died by hanging if it is not an insane person.

We see from the preceding list that female trigrams indicate curses from a variety of unfortunate ghosts, such as women who died before their time or in childbirth or people who suffered accidents or capital punishment. Shamans were sources of witchcraft just as deceased mothers were of curses. Portals and passageways in built spaces were also dangerous. Most interesting for our purposes is the curse under the trigram Xun, which involves the premature death of a woman in childbirth (here written as *zi* 字 *mə-dzə-a, the verbal form of the word "child" *zi* 子 *tsə?). If the extraordinary male numeral of a 9 appears, then the curse might come from a woman who died in a traumatic birth involving multiple births, much like the mother of the Chu progenitor in the *Chu ju*. As we saw earlier, the Xun trigram was associated with spring and the rebirth of the moon. If a potent male number was combined with the strong female trigram, then the curse may have come from one who died due to an *excess* of fertility.

This type of condition seems to be mentioned only in Chu or Chu-influenced texts as far as we know. The word *la* 柆 (*r̥ˤəp) used in the preceding Xun curse list is explained in the *Shuowen* dictionary as "to split word" (*zhemu* 折木). Other ways of writing this word included the more common *xie* 脅 *qʰ<r>ep as in *xiesheng*, "split-side birth." The *Chu ju* text used a loan word *la* 臘 *rˤəp. Notably the link between shamans and "splitting" is reflected in the later *Shuogua* text attached as a commentary to the *Zhouyi*. In a section that lists the mantic images associated with the Dui (female) trigram, it says:

兌為澤，為少女，為巫，為口舌，為毀折，為附決
Dui is (associated with) still water, younger daughters, shamans, mouth and tongue, smashing and splitting, dropping and bursting.

The images associated with the Xun in the *Shuogua* do not include shamans or childbirth, although perhaps we see a reflection of the large-headed demon that frightened a girl to death listed under the Dui trigram in the *Shifa*. Also interesting is that Dui in the *Shifa* is linked to White and the West, not Xun:

巽為木，為風，為長女，為繩直，為工，為白，為長，為高，為進退，為不果，為臭．其於人也，為寡髮，為廣顙，為多白眼．
The Xun is (associated with) wood, wind, the eldest girl, the plumb line, the carpenter's square, white, length, altitude, moving forward and backward, no results, and smells. Its (manifestation) in people is baldness, broad foreheads, excessive revealing of the whites of the eyes.

Kun in the *Shuogua* is associated with "mothers" as in the *Shifa* but also the color black, which in the *Shifa* was linked to Li.

坤為地，為母，為布，為釜，為吝嗇，為均，為子母牛，為大輿，為文，為眾，為柄，其於地也為黑．
Kun is (associated with) earth, mothers, cloth, measuring vessels, stinginess, tools for leveling (dirt), female calves, large carriages, patterns, multitudes, handles; and black due to its (connection to) Earth.

Although the Li trigram is accorded the association with the middle daughter 中 in the family hierarchy and a "large abdomen" (*dafu* 大腹) in the *Shuogua*, all the imagery is mostly Yang in nature and the curious obverse to the qualities assigned to the middle brother, Kan, which are mostly Yin (Water, ditches, concealment, etc.). This is not the case in the *Shifa* where Kan is associated with Fire and Li with Water. By the time the material compiled into the *Shuogua* was attached to the *Zhouyi*, the immediacy of the "images" as potential sources of curses or as supernatural manifestations seems to be lost.

Beside natural earthly manifestations of supernatural influence indicated by the female trigrams, by the third centuries BCE, astral influences are increasingly noted. There is mention of a multiple birth in the "Stars" 星 section of the Shuihudi *Day Book*. This section explains which of the twenty-eight celestial lodges (*su* 宿) were considered auspicious or inauspicious for human activity. It notes that the "Eastern Well" 東井 star was bad for everything, including marriage and birthing. Not only would a woman be subject to birthing multiples 多子, but any baby born on a day dominated by the Well lodge would die within ten days.[29] In later texts the Well lodge (signified by either star γ Geminorum or μ Geminorum) was associated with an area of the sky linked to the Qin state. However, this must have been a Han attempt to link Qin to an inauspicious star, since it is unlikely that the Qin-period Shuihudi almanac would follow this. Generally, it seemed that astronomers watched the movement of these stars across the sky and the travel of visible planets into particular lodges and calculated their auspiciousness according to the phases of the moon, the season, or to the ten sun/stem signs as indicated by the rotation of the dipper handle on divinatory instruments, an astrolabe called *shipan* 式盤. Other baleful lodges for children include "Carriage Ghost" 輿鬼, indicating their forthcoming illness, and Yi 翼, predicating that they might become shamans.[30] We saw the negative influence of shamans in the *Shifa* curses. Apparently, becoming a shaman was something decided by cosmic influences and beyond parental control.

In the *Day Books*, stars, ritual calendar day signs, and the Yin or Yang strength of each day could affect the delivery of the child and whether it survives. Most dangerous for newborns were the ghosts of other babies that died before they could walk. They could cause unsuccessful deliveries and the death of other infants. The best protection for an infant was to be conceived on auspicious days of the calendar and nurtured *in utero* in an environment devoid of negative influences such as thunder.[31] A similar approach appears in the Han *Taichan shu*. The pregnant woman's environment was controlled to avoid contact with visual images or foods that could affect the gender or health of the fetus, such as dwarves, monkeys, and pungent foods with inauspicious images such as onions and ginger (which could result in excessive branching of appendages such as an extra finger or toe), or rabbit meat (which could result in a child with a cleft lip). The gender of the fetus could be affected by the mother's "inner imaging to complete the child," particularly during the third month of pregnancy.[32] Where and when the afterbirth was buried could affect the woman's next pregnancy, the ease of the delivery, as well as the gender of the baby; hence, a diviner capable of calculating a combined system of geomancy and time calculation had to be consulted. Certain foods could affect the delivery. For example, an "easy delivery" (*yichu* 易出) would occur if the woman ate the head of a white male dog (*bai mugou shou* 白牡狗首).³³ Postnatal precautions were also indicated. As soon as the child was born, it was covered with special dirt and then bathed. The mother then drank some of the bathwater to protect herself from later ailments.

Sequestering

By the Han period of early imperial China, when theories of a gendered universe became accepted doctrine, ritual texts make clear the need to sequester birthing females. Earlier records suggest a similar anxiety. Generally, during the Han time, we know that Yin *qi* was associated with fluid, the body, earth, the dark moon, and death, and a spiritual essence called *po* 魄. This was counterbalanced with Yang *qi* associated with air, identity (*ming* 名), consciousness (*zhi* 知), heaven, bright light, and birth, and a spiritual essence called *hun* 魂. The bodily fluids along with the afterbirth belonged to the Po category and therefore had to be managed carefully. Diviners queried the powers over whether a woman would leak during her pregnancy.³⁴

In a record possibly dating to the time earlier than the *Chu ju*, we learn that women about to give birth were sequestered together, left to announce the births only after they were all over. A tale preserved in the *Zuozhuan* about events in 513 BCE concerns two potential heirs born to mothers in the same family and sequestered together:³⁵

> 公衍、公為之生也，其母偕出，公衍先生，公為之母曰："相與偕出." 請相與偕告. 三日，公為生，其母先以告，公為為兄.
> When Gong Yan and Gong Wei were born, their mothers were sent out together. Gong Yan was born first, but Gong Wei's mother suggested to the other woman that they announce the births together. But after three days when Gong Wei was born, his mother went ahead and announced his birth first. As a result, Gong Wei was considered the elder brother.

It is not clear what type of environment that the women gave birth in, but it was clearly outside of the regular home. In Han-period ritual records, elite women near the end of their terms stayed in "side rooms" (*ceshi* 側室) to assure auspicious births.³⁶ This room was most likely behind one of the chambers in the women's quarters. It is clear in this account that the birthing time was considered one of great vulnerability to spiritual contamination, particularly between the mother, child, and father. Contact between the parents was strictly controlled, with the mother and baby kept hidden from the father until after the birth and after they had both fully bathed. Before then, only a nursemaid was allowed access to the mother. From the Han-edited ritual text, the *Ritual Records*:

妻將生子, 及月辰, 居側室. 夫使人日再問之. 作而自問之, 妻不敢見, 使姆衣服而對. 至於子生, 夫復使人日再問之. 夫齊, 則不入側室之門. 子生, 男子設弧於門左, 女子設帨於門右. 三日始負子, 男射女否.

When a wife was going to give birth, as she neared her time, she lived in a side room. The husband sent someone to ask after her twice each day. After the wife felt that the child was coming out, he would ask after her himself, but the wife dared not look at him, sending a nursemaid with just clothing as an answer. Once the child began to arrive, the husband again sent someone to ask after her twice each day. While the husband performed purification rituals, he would not enter the door of the side room. Once the child was born, if it was a boy, a wooden bow would be set on the left side of the door; if it was a girl, a cloth belt was set on the right side of the door. After three days, the child could begin to be carried. Boys practice archery but girls do not.

Shang ritual records dated to the King Wu Ding period suggest a need to sequester birthing women. Records show that some women stayed at a place outside the city with the name "Child Citadel," Zijing 子京 written together as a single graph. Although most inscriptions with this place-name are fragmentary (and *zi* might have referred to the royal Shang lineage name, the Child, rather than simply a "child"), we see a concern with distress occurring there in the divination records. Questions concern the issue of whether one or another member of the royal couple—the queen or even in some cases the king—should go to Zijing, and whether a successful birth would occur there. Although difficult births were not specified, sometimes curses had to be exorcised using a *liao* 燎 fire sacrifice or female ancestor spirits called upon for special aid.[37]

In the *Chu ju* text, the first site of rule for the Chu ancestors was called the "Citadel Ancestral Shrine," the Jingzong 京宗. This is the site that the founder ancestor and his mate occupied and presumably where the next generation was born. In the ideology of the *Chu ju*, this site was associated with the birth of a people as well as a political identity. Like the earlier Shang records, the text reveals a concern with smooth versus difficult birthing experiences. But the fact that it was a traumatic birthing experience that resulted in the Chu people reveals the purposeful Chu alignment with a non-Zhou alterity that will be discussed more fully in chapter 5.

In the discussion of the words "to birth" in chapter 1, we mentioned the idea of an enclosed space possibly associated with the process. Two types of enclosed spaces are mentioned in the *Chu ju* and, although neither was marked as specifically for birthing, they can provide hints as to the Chu idea of sacred built environments. The first mentioned is the "Citadel Ancestral Shrine," Jingzong, where founder ancestor Ji Lian and his wife, a Shang princess (also symbolic of a purposeful alignment with a non-Zhou history), lived.[38] This shrine was associated with the auspicious birth of twins. It was also where founder Xue Yin (possibly the same as the legendary Yu Xiong), the father of a second set of twins (the latter one tragically born), visited before the birth. Some scholars suggest that the first part of the name of the place, *jing* 京 ("citadel, capital," *kraŋ), was a Chu dialect loan for *jing* 荊 ("thorny," *krəŋ), one of the alternative names applied to the Chu people. While this is hard to prove, we do know from the record of the second traumatic birthing tale that thorns were used in the process.[39] This will be discussed in more detail in chapter 6.

Other scholars claim that Jingzong referred to the ancestral Zhou capital, "Citadel Hao Ancestral Zhou Shrine" (Haojing Zong Zhou 鎬京宗周), since the Han-period historical record, the *Shiji*, recorded that Yu Xiong had served the Zhou king around this time.[40] In Zhou birth legends, the birth of a founder was trouble free, so perhaps an association with the legend of the founder working in Zhou would be considered auspicious. But it is unclear why a Shang princess would go to a Zhou capital (and presumably generations before the Zhou conquest of the Shang). Also, the Zhou capital was referred to as either Haojing or Zong Zhou, not as Jingzong, so the actual site of Jingzong (if there was an actual site), which would seem to include a primary ancestral shrine (*zong*), remains a mystery.

The second sacred enclosure mentioned in the *Chu ju* was linked to a sacrificial ritual to accompany geomantic divination concerning moving and creating a capital. The spiritual object of the divination was likely an ancestor spirit, the divinity Ji Lian or perhaps the legendary founder Yu Xiong. According to the *Chu ju*, generations of the earliest Chu rulers up to Xiong Yi (aka Yin Yi 酓繹) lived in Jingzong. But Xiong Yi (sometime in the early Western Zhou period, during the tenth century BCE) found it necessary to move the people to a place named "Yi Mound," Yitun 夷屯, perhaps another name for Yiling 夷陵, a settlement probably located north of the Dan River and known generally as Danyang 丹陽, a former Manyi 蠻夷 (southern non-Zhou peoples) territory (according to the *Shiji*).[41] According to the *Chu ju*, this move required divination and a sacrifice involving the construction of a sacred enclosure. This enclosure, believed by some scholars to be a type of ancestral shrine, was called a Pian-wood Room 楩室, also read as "Comfort room" 便室.[42] Modern scholar Chen Wei suspects that this sacred room might have been somewhat like the "Closed-off Chamber" (*bigong* 閟宮), which as we discussed earlier may have been used as a Gaomei fertility ritual site.[43] The first stanza of the ode on this chamber in the *Book of Odes* celebrates Jiang Yuan giving birth in the "Closed-off Chamber" (see chapter 2) and the last stanza describes a multiroom building made with different types of wood and an ornamental roof.

One signature of the sanctification of the chamber in the *Chu ju* was the placement of the corpse of a young calf inside it. If we think of this act in iconographic terms, it could be represented by the oracle bone graph for "home" (*jia* 家) (see chart 4). The *Chu ju* emphasizes the timing of the sacrifice in order to explain a special Chu term for sacrifice (written with a variant of "night" 夜 made up of sematic signifiers of the graph for "evening," *xi* 夕 over that for "divinity" 示, and read as a variant of "sacrifice" *ji* 祭) that was also used in terms for the first three months of spring (at the beginning of the Chu calendar).[44] The *Chu*

Chart 4. Sequestering images

Shang Zijing

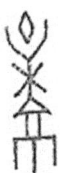 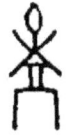

Shang Building with a Pig ("home" 家)

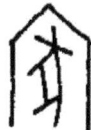

ju does not mention the use of the term but emphasizes the need for secrecy. The young sacrificial animal (perhaps a specially raised *lao* 牢?) had to be "stolen" from a people that had long been absorbed into the Chu state and "secretly" inserted into the enclosure at night. The name of the people, the Ruo 鄀, is linked in another version of Chu origins associated with the mountain where a deity (not called Ji Lian, but Changyi 昌意) first descended. In the *Chu ju*, the diviner who officiated this Chu rite was also named Ruo.[45] The *Chu ju* notes:

> 至酓繹與屈紃, 思（使）鄀嗌卜徙於夷屯（夷陵）, 爲楩（便?）室, 室既成, 無以內之, 乃竊鄀人之犝以祭。懼其宝（主）, 夜而內尸, 氐（抵）今日楑, 楑必夜。
>
> When it came to the time of Yin Yi and Qu Xun, they had Ruo Yi divine about moving to Yitun and then created a Pian-room. After the room was finished, they had nothing to put in it, so they stole a calf from the Ruo people to sacrifice. Fearing (discovery by) the owner, they waited until night to put the corpse into (the room). Hence, today this is called "sacrifice," as "sacrifice" must be at night.

The illicit nature of this sacrifice performed with a stolen animal at night emphasizes the Yin nature of this rite. It also forms the communal bond of a shared secret.[46] Notably, this built enclosure could not be penetrated without the bloodied body of a freshly killed baby animal—a visual experience that seems almost like birthing in reverse: the return of a sacrificial baby animal to the original womb-like enclosure. The need to provide captured game to consecrate a site may trace back to early hunting and covenant rituals. There was also a tradition of sacrificing an animal at the resolution of lawsuits, although in this case, the ritual officers and plaintiffs belonged to the same people.[47] The *Chu ju* recasts old tales into a new version of myth, secularizing old rites. Just as it feels the need to explain the origin of the "Thorn" people, it attempts to explain the "Night" sacrifice. It explains that the body of the animal was chosen simply to "have something to put in the enclosure" and that it was done at night only to escape the notice of the Ruo people. It is unclear whether animal blood was considered as dangerous as female birthing fluids or even if this ritual, certainly involving some kind of spirits, had any conscious association with birthing or heritage. The fact that the rite was not performed in the main ancestral hall in Jingzong, but in a separate and secret location, perhaps associated with an earlier burial, suggests a type of symbolic sequestering.

A Question of Thorns

The birth of Xue Yin's (or Yu Xiong's) heir initiated the era of successful Chu sociopolitical reproduction. The Chu state by the time of King Dao 悼 (r. 384–381 BCE), the last leader mentioned in the *Chu ju*, had been flourishing for centuries. Sequestering birthing women no doubt was practiced. The only symbol of the ancient birthing mother's location in the *Chu ju* was the presence of thorns and their use by a shaman practitioner. In a later text found in the old Qi region of the northeast, thorns had a negative association. They caused the depletion of *de* energy, a phenomenon called "slicing, punishment" (*xing* 刑).[48] In the *Day Books*, thorn knives and arrows were used to chase away demonic influences. The *Zuozhuan* (Zhao 12) record of Spring and Autumn court activities mentions the use of peach-wood shafts with thorn arrowheads for exorcism.[49] The "Jiaosi zhi" 郊祀志 chapter of the *Qian Hanshu* 前漢書 notes that "male thorns" were used to make poles for a banner with the Sun and Moon, the North Pole, and the Rising Dragon (constellation) painted on it (*yi mujing hua fan, riyue beidou denglong* 以牡荆畫幡, 日月北斗登龍). Male thorns may also have been employed in fertility rituals (see chapter 2). Basically, a male thorn is one that does not produce seeds. It could be cut when the moon had a halo around it and used to make a wrap for those endangered by illness.[50] Because the verb used for the operation with the thorn in the *Chu ju* could be loaned for many similar words, there is controversy as to exactly what the thorn was used for. Some say it was a cutting instrument, others a sewing instrument, and others even suggest that the skin of thorn branches was used to wrap wounds on either the baby or the mother after the emergency surgery to get the heir out. Doctors in later time periods used sharp objects to prod the baby into turning around during breach births.[51] Thorns were also used in magical rituals to "confront" demons as if in a judicial trial. Any of these explanations might fit the text, which we will discuss in more detail in chapters 5 and 6.

The *Chu ju* text does not reflect the power of stars or other natural forces but instead reverts to the power of legendary ancestors. Unlike the Baoshan divination text, there was no record of temporal influences, although recording the spatial locations (the "residences," *ju* 居) of the originating ancestral pairs and the subsequent generations of rulers was clearly as important as listing their names.[52] The ritual use of a text like the *Chu ju* was certainly different from that of the stalk divination texts, although divination is mentioned regarding the establishment of the first Chu capital.

Ancient records preserve for us prayers, legends, and divination guides concerned with birthing in ancient China. The mother was the vehicle for the perpetuation of civilization. She was the cosmic portal for the renewal of human life and the barrier most close to the state of death and eternity. It is no surprise then to find in a literary record dominated by men's affairs also a focus on controlling fertility, marriage, and birth. Legends connect the strongest male supernatural powers with the birth of founders, but at times the strong male cosmic agents have disastrous consequences on a woman's health, splitting her open with an overabundance of offspring. Balance then seemed to be the harbinger of a healthy society.

5

Divine Origins and Chu Genealogical History

Most early Chinese genealogical records of the birth and history of a people consist of a series of ancestral names, assumed by most to be male, one "begetting" or "producing" (*sheng* 生 or *chan* 產) another over the course of the Three Dynasties (*sandai* 三代, Xia, Shang, and Zhou). This type of historical record, found in the *Shiji* 史記, the *Shiben* 世本, or *Da Dai Liji* 大戴禮記, date to the Han period, and, generally, seem compiled of earlier materials arranged to fit with popular cosmology. They subscribe to a hagiography of cosmic progenitors that became popular around the same time as the Yin Yang Wuxing scheme of natural philosophy at the end of the Warring States period, although with an added imperialist twist: there was only one supreme emperor-like god that all lineages descended from.[1] In this scheme, the Chu people descended from the Yellow Emperor (Huangdi 黃帝), an ancestral deity mentioned earliest in a northeastern regional inscription associated with the Tian 田 group that took over the state of Qi during the middle Warring States period (the Chen Hou Yinzi *dui* 陳侯因資敦, see the following discussion). Huangdi did not feature in Warring States–period Chu texts at all.

The *Chu ju* reveals a pre-imperial layer of genealogical writing. Unlike later genealogical histories that tend to secularize ancient gods, the *Chu ju* focuses on divine origins and the geomantic significance of places occupied by rulers with particular names. The tone of the initial tale of divine origins shares the same religious sense of the supernatural as the *Shanhaijing* and *Chuci*. The most distant ancestor mentioned in the *Chu ju*, Ji Lian 季連, like Changyi 昌意, Zhu Rong 祝融, and other spirits, was not born but "descended" (*jiang* 降).² Instead of tracing one's ancestry back to the first one who served a Zhou king as in Western Zhou bronze inscriptions, the Chu text traces it back to immortal deities. That the earthly incarnations of these spirits were considered temporary or a matter of heavenly arbitration (or "command," *ming* 命) is further suggested in the *Chu ju* when the woman who tragically died giving birth to the Chu progenitor then "went to visit Heaven" (*bin yu tian* 賓於天).³ The inclusion of an ancestral mother figure also links the *Chu ju* origin myth to other accounts that include birth mothers.

Archaeological evidence unquestionably supports the textual evidence for a firmly established patriarchy in ancient China. Hence, the assumption that all lineage heads—no matter how unconventional their names—were male is well founded. A question arises however concerning the identities of some mythical founder figures, particularly ones for whom there is no textual documentation until millennia after their presumed existences. They seem less "historical" personas than god-kings, perhaps contemporaneous (often supernaturally charged) emblems of peoples' attempts to carve a historical identity out of a chaotic world in which the legitimacy of earlier Zhou-inspired powerful lineages had collapsed. For peoples originally on the fringes of the Zhou world, such as the Chu, this issue may have been particularly keen. With regard to the personas in the beginning, and most mythical, section of the *Chu ju*, we analyze two related issues. One involves the role of the ancestress in birthing the Chu people/nation and the second the possible gender-bending connotations underlying the names used for the presumed male founders.

First, given the respect for lineage hierarchy associated with ancestor worship in ancient China, we should understand that worship of powerful female ancestors was generally in association with their reproductive roles and the powerful patriarchs with whom they were associated. Lengthy middle- and late-period Western Zhou inscriptions from the Fufeng region, which trace multiple generations of powerful lineage heads, such as on the Shi Qiang *pan* 史牆盤 and the recently recovered Lai 逨 bronzes, mention no women at all. On the other hand, hundreds of marriage inscriptions and dedications to particular "mothers" (probably dead) on bronze sacrificial vessels acknowledge the critical role of the female to lineage history during the Western Zhou and Spring and Autumn periods. Earlier, during the late Shang period, women who were worshipped for their power included Fu Hao 婦好, mate of King Wu Ding 武丁. Her shrine-topped lavish tomb was discovered in Anyang in 1976, and her tomb was filled with iconography possibly associated with fertility. Later, bronze inscriptions mention the occasional queen, such as early Western Zhou–period Wang Jiang 王姜 or the early Spring and Autumn–period Jin Jiang 晉姜, both of whom command, but seemingly only when their husbands were absent. The power of mother spirits is confirmed in the mid–Western Zhou inscription on the Dong *ding* 彧鼎 (also from the Fufeng region). Dong's mother responded to his prayer for protection when he went off to battle.[4]

By the time of the late Spring and Autumn period in eastern regions, we begin to find some acknowledgment of female ancestors in lineage history, such as in the Shu Yi 叔夷 bell inscriptions of the fifth-century BCE state of Qi 齊, or its satellite nations of Ju 莒 and Chen 陳.[5] Unfortunately, Chu bronze inscriptions, like the majority of later bronze inscriptions, did not name any ancestral spirits, so it is difficult to know if female spirits were included in their annual feasts. The fourth-century BCE bamboo divination texts of Baoshan and Xin Cai likewise seem to favor male spirits. Only the influence from the recently deceased mothers were deemed potent, and even then they received fewer sacrificial bribes than the fathers. It is likely that, by the third century BCE when the *Chu ju* was circulated and the notion of a gendered cosmos was beginning to become popular, powerful female progenitors and nature goddesses, such as the female version of Taiyi, Nüwa, or Xi Wangmu 西王母, "Grandmother of the West," had already started to transplant the female ancestor spirits of earlier lineages. The earliest reference to it is in the Chu Silk Manuscript, where Nüwa along with Fuxi gives birth to the cosmos much along the lines of what is credited to Taiyi in the text *Taiyi sheng shui*. But, as in the *Chu ju*, the Chu Silk Manuscript's account involved two sets of twins, but these evolved into abstract aspects of the cosmos such as seasons and so forth rather than specifically named ancestors. By the early imperial period, Nüwa became associated with fertility and parturition.[6] Xi Wangmu, on the other hand, served as the conduit back into the land of immortals and spirits. She was associated with the transcendence of time rather than the birth of it, the Daoist reversal from living rather than its creator.[7] The association of female goddesses with the birth of the cosmos and the "return" of immortals to the void fits with the Daoist idea of "mother" discussed in chapter 3.

As part of our analysis of the ancestral spirits listed in the *Chu ju*, we will compare them with the spirits mentioned in the Chu genealogies provided in the transmitted texts.[8] First, we shall consider the figure of Huangdi, which by the Han period had become the ultimate founder spirit. Although we cannot be sure the first mention of the name Huangdi has anything to do with the Han period founder-god, we note that the name was first applied to an ancient ancestor by the mid–Warring States Qi king, Wei Yingqi 齊威王嬰齊 (r. 378–320 BCE). He reigned right around the time period that the tales reflected in the *Chu ju* were probably circulating. For King Wei, his distant ancestor was a royal ancestor spirit associated with the Tian 田 (*lˤiŋ) lineage, which had descended from the earlier state of Chen (*lriŋ) (a near homophone), a small eastern state located during the Spring and Autumn period between the powerful states of Chu and Qi and alternately occupied by one or the other. He referred to Huangdi as a high ancestor or founder (*gaozu* 高祖) and prayed to him for protection of the Qi state. This Huangdi was the most ancient member of a pantheon of ancestors that extended through time to King Wei's own "Brilliant deceased-father," *huangkao* 皇考.[9]

The title Huangdi would have had an archaic ring to it when read aloud. Since the name Huang, "yellow" (黃 *N-kʷˤaŋ), was phonically similar to the standard Zhou epithet meaning "great, awe-inspiring," or "brilliant" applied to the most distant ancestors (*huang* 皇 *Gʷˤaŋ). By the Middle Western Zhou period, the word "yellow" is found in bronze inscriptions as a proper noun and as a color. As a color word, it could refer to something made of metal or to the color of the hair of older people. The term "yellowed aged-ones" (*huanggou* 黃耉) was a reference to elders and ancestors. The ancient words for "yellowed aged-ones" and "brilliant deceased-father" were near homophones. It is unlikely that King Wei knew that the title "god" *di* 帝 had been applied by the Shang royalty in that region to their dead fathers over half a millennium earlier. By his time, it was a title applied to many legendary prehistoric kings as well as to Shangdi in the sky and various mountain spirits. It is possibly that the title Huangdi did not originally refer to a single deity but was in fact a group term for the many distant founder ancestors (just as Yu during the Shang was a term applied to many recent founder ancestors, the opposite of *huang*). If the term was common in states to the south of Qi and east of the ancient Chen area, the Han dynasty founder's homeland, perhaps that might help explain how it came to represent the ultimate founder ancestor. This area was also occupied by the Chu royal family before being crushed by Qin in 223 BCE, so although the early Han founder had an association with late Chu culture, it was only as a veneer over his native eastern culture.

Han genealogical histories tracing Chu ancestry include a number of spirits not mentioned in the *Chu ju*. Most begin with the descended spirit "Fine Intention," Changyi 昌意. The *Da Dai Liji* and *Shiben* versions also generally include wives at this stage of social reproduction, using language similar to that found in the *Chu ju*. Wives were provided for Huangdi, Changyi, and Gaoyang shi 高陽氏 (the High Yang clan, another name for the god Zhuanxu 顓頊)[10] in the main lineage trunk and also for some specific to the Chu branch, such as Lao Tong and Lu Zhong 陸終 (another name for Zhu Rong). The *Shiji* generally does not include the female counterparts in its history of the Chu royal family (the "Chu shijia" 楚世家 chapter) but does include similar style pairings for prehistorical god-kings Huangdi, Changyi, and Zhuanxu in its "Wudi benji" 五帝本紀 chapter. The information and names vary only slightly among the different Han records suggesting that these were commonly known tales. However, in some cases the names were transcribed using different characters that were either similar in sound or graphic style, suggesting that while the tales were well known, they had different paths of transmission, some oral and some written. This reflects back in time to the different names for the Three Chu Progenitors evident in Warring States documents. Indeed, we find different names for the Three in the transmitted texts. The graphs for Lao Tong were misread as Juan Zhang 卷章. Zhu Rong was written down as Lu Zhong or Chong Li but also explained as a title held by various prehistorical god-kings. Some claim Yu Xiong was another name either for Ji Lian himself, for his offspring, Xue Xiong, or for Xue Xiong's offspring.

The *Shanhaijing* adds supernatural twists to the pairings of god-kings with ancestress/birth mothers. For example, Changyi was born of Huangdi's wife, who was named Leizu 嫘祖 in the "Wudi benji" and elsewhere, in the *Shanhaijing*, was called "Thunder Ancestor" (Leizu 雷祖).[11] Both texts record that Changyi then "descended" (to the Ruo River 若水), but the *Shanhaijing* gives Changyi another son, Han Liu 韓流, who took as wife a "Daughter of the Mud People" (淖子) named Anü 阿女, who then produced Zhuanxu.[12] In the *Shiji*, Changyi married a child/daughter (*zi* 子) of the people of the Shu Mountains 蜀山氏, named Chang Pu 昌僕. In another example, we find three somewhat similar graphs in different tales for the names of the young woman of the Guifang people (鬼方氏之妹) who married Lu Zhong: Kui 嬇, Tui 隤, or Zi 瀆. Scholars from the Fudan University Excavated Text and Paleography Research Center have pointed out that versions of the tale, found in the *Shiben*, *Da Dai Liji*, the *Fengsu tongyi*, and the *Hanshu*, all have different variations of the same word for the name of the birth mother but all mean "to split open."[13] The child was Ji Lian, who appears at the beginning of the *Chu ju* version.

The history of the Chu people in *Shiji* chapter 40, the "Chu shijia" 楚世家, includes many figures not in the *Chu ju* version. The lineages of god-kings leading up the Chu founder also differ. In the "Chu shijia" the god-king Zhuanxu Gaoyang is the branch of Huangdi's descendants that start the Chu house. There are two accounts preserved of Zhuanxu Gaoyang's ancestors and their female partners:

The "Wudi benji" 五帝本紀 chapter of the *Shiji* has:[14]

嫘祖為黃帝正妃, 生二子, 其後皆有天下: . . . 其二曰昌意, 降居若水. 昌意娶蜀山氏女, 曰昌僕, 生高陽, 高陽有聖德焉.
Leizu was Huangdi's principal wife. She had two sons who later ruled the world. . . . The second one was called Changyi. He descended to live in the Ruo River region. Changyi took a girl of the Shu Mountain people, called Chang Pu. She gave birth to Gaoyang. Gaoyang got his sagely virtue thereby.

The *Shiben* has a similar variation:[15]

黃帝娶于西陵氏之子, 謂之纍祖, 產青陽及昌意. 昌意娶于濁山氏之子, 謂之昌僕, 生顓頊.
Huangdi took a child of the Xiling people as wife, called Leizu. She produced Qingyang and Changyi. Changyi took as wife a child of the Zhuo Mountain people, called Chang Pu. She gave birth to Zhuanxu.

In the "Chu shijia" 楚世家 account, after a series of "begets" (X *sheng* Y, Y *sheng* Z, in which all are presumably male), we come to a split-side birthing tale resulting in multiple births. Ji Lian is the last of six kids. In this tale, Lu Zhong 陸終, not his wife, "begets" the children. While hagiographies that include or exclude female figures suggest different mythical or regional narrative strategies, some more or less similar to the *Chu ju*, none of these include the same level of birthing detail, suggesting perhaps later censorship of the early tales. Words and figures important to understanding the *Chu ju* account, repeated in the following with detailed annotation, are in bold and underlined for emphasis.

The *Shiji* account of the origins of the Chu people:[16]

楚之先祖出自帝<u>顓頊高陽</u>. 高陽者, <u>黃帝</u>之孫, 昌意之子也. 高陽生稱, 稱生卷章, 卷章生<u>重黎</u>.
<u>重黎</u>為帝嚳高辛居火正, 甚有功, 能光融天下, 帝嚳命曰祝融. 共工氏作亂, 帝嚳使重黎誅之而不盡. 帝乃以庚寅日誅重黎, 而以其

弟吳回為重黎後，復居火正，為祝融。
吳回生陸終。陸終生子六人，坼剖而產焉。其長一曰昆吾；二曰參胡；三曰彭祖；四曰會人；五曰曹姓；六曰季連，羋姓，楚其後也。昆吾氏，夏之時嘗為侯伯，桀之時湯滅之。彭祖氏，殷之時嘗為侯伯，殷之末世滅彭祖氏。
季連生附沮，附沮生穴熊。其后中微，或在中國，或在蠻夷，弗能紀其世。周文王之時，季連之苗裔曰鬻熊。
鬻熊子事文王，蚤卒。其子曰熊麗。熊麗生熊狂，熊狂生熊繹。熊繹當周成王之時，舉文、武勤勞之後嗣，而封熊繹於楚蠻，封以子男之田，姓羋氏，居丹陽。

The founder ancestor of the Chu came from Deity Zhuanxu, the High Yang, who was the grandson of **Huangdi** and the son of Changyi. The High Yang begat Cheng who begat Juanzhang who begat **Chong Li**.

Chong Li resided (in the position of) Fire Regulator for Deity Ku, earning a lot of merit and bringing radiance to All Under Heaven, so Deity Ku called him "Invoker Smelter" (Zhu Rong). When Chief Gonggong rebelled, Deity Ku sent Chong Li to exterminate him, but Chong Li was unsuccessful, so the Deity terminated Chong Li on a Gengyin day. Then his younger brother Wuhui acted as Chong Li's descendant and took over the position of Fire Regulator and the name Invoker Smelter.

Wuhui begat **Lu Zhong, who begat six children who were born from him in a split-side manner.** His eldest was Kunwu, second Canhu, third Pengzu, fourth the Hui people, fifth the Cao lineage, and sixth **Ji Lian's Mi lineage from whom the Chu descend.** The chiefs of the Kunwu often acted as officials during the Xia period, but during Jie's reign they were exterminated by Tang. The chiefs of Pengzu often acted as officials during the Yin period, but were wiped out when the Yin fell.

Ji Lian begat Fu Ju, who begat **Xue Xiong**, whose descendants from this point on thinned out, some being in the Central States and others with the Manyi peoples, so there is no record of his lineage. During the time of King Wen of Zhou, the descendant of **Ji Lian** was called **Yu Xiong**. Yu Xiong's son served King Wen but died early. His son was called **Xiong Li**. Xiong Li begat Xiong Kuang, who begat Xiong Yi. During Zhou King Cheng's time, because Xiong Yi aided King Cheng and was the descendant of ancestors who worked hard for Kings Wen and Wu, he was granted cultivated fields to rule with the rank of *zinan* (the lowest of the five political ranks) among the Man people of Chu with the lineage name Mi. He resided at Danyang.

In the *Chu ju* version, there is no Lu Zhong. The father of the Chu people is a descendant of Ji Lian's, called Xue Yin. His wife, a woman named Lie 列, "Break Apart," experienced the split-side birth. Ji Lian was the ultimate founder not Huangdi or Zhuanxu. He was Heaven-descended and not one of multiple children born out of a woman's side.[17] Although we cannot say that the *Chu ju* was a manual used for mantic purposes, like the *Shifa* or *Day Books*, it was not a secular history either. The standard narrative of a state's origins and its royal lineage found in Han histories is completely ignored in the *Chu ju*. It includes figures and bits of legend familiar from the later histories, but the names are somewhat different and it skips entirely many of the earliest names listed in the transmitted texts, while at the same time adding new content. How universal this Chu narrative was we do not know.

The birth of the Chu people required the descent of a spirit, marriage and birth, and finally death of the mother. In the *Chu ju*, two contrasting birthing experiences, one auspicious and one tragic, each producing twins, represented the social reproduction of the people. Once the Chu identity was created and the sacred enclosure consecrated, the text becomes a patriarchal history of royal ancestor spirits and their migrations from one Chu "dwelling, residence, political social center" (*ju* 居) to another. Since the location of the king in ancient times was often the rhetoric used to anchor an event in time when making a historical record, this text may have served as a reference work for the ritual archivists (*shi* 史 or *yin* 尹).[18] The initial section of the text focusing on divine origins suggests also a role for the text in storytelling. This latter role makes sense when we consider the larger context of birth lore and later Han redactions of the birth tales of early founders. This is particularly true of the magical "split-side" births (which we will discuss at length in the next chapter).

The descended divinity in the *Chu ju* was named Ji Lian, a figure that also appears in transmitted genealogies. The *Chu ju* version is unique. In it, like many god-kings in the *Shanhaijing*, he first arrived on a mountaintop. There he lived in a cave until he heard about a Shang princess who wanted to get married and was wandering around a mountain (possibly practicing the Gaomei fertility rite). He traveled up a river and married her. According to the *Chu ju*, this princess was the daughter of a legendary Shang king who is known in other accounts for wandering from place to place, leading his people tirelessly to find exactly the right place to build a capital. He is credited with being the first king who established the capital at Anyang, which is known now by the Zhou term as the "Wastes of Yin," Yinxu 殷墟. After meeting Ji Lian, the princess, named Ancestress Wei, gave birth to twins and they settled in the first ancestral site called Jingzong.

After a gap of an unknown number of generations, the next Chu ruler mentioned is Xue Yin, whose name is discussed in chapter 1. He was the third deity in the list of the Three Chu Progenitors in the fourth-century BCE Chu divination records (the name Ji Lian does not appear in those texts). In the *Chu ju*, Xue Yin visited the ancestral site and received a bride, Ancestress Split (or Li Ghost?), whose subsequent birthing of twins was only halfway successful. The second child refused to come down the birth canal but burst out of her side. We see this type of birth in other non-Zhou myth cycles, which will be discussed in the next chapter. In the *Chu ju* version, a shaman-midwife attended the birth. This shaman used a thorn (or a bunch of thorns) to perform some sort of medical procedure on her. The name of this shaman appears in *Chuci* and the *Shanhaijing* as the descended spirit, Wu Xian 巫咸, who according to myth was active during the Shang period.[19] It seems that the ancestress no longer could use her human body after its side was split open. (As readers, we can visualize the side of a silkworm cocoon, mentioned in the quote from Xunzi in chapter 3.) The *Chu ju* explains that she went to "visit" Heaven, suggesting that she would be back again later, perhaps in another form. It seems that the Chu people at least envisioned their female and male ancestors as immortals both occupying space up in the sky.

The point by the *Chu ju* writers of describing this last scene was to explain the magical origins of the Chu birth and name. This is the only example in such tales where it is the manner of healing that determined the name. In *Zuozhuan* birth tales, which also focus on naming, the names might derive from birthmarks or other physical or behavioral attributes of the infants, but details about the mother's body and birthing experience are completely absent.[20] Whenever an infant was described in the *Zuozhuan*, it was invariably because some detail was predictive of the fate of the infant in the role of a future ruler or contender for the throne. One can imagine an early *Day Book* for interpreting birthmarks and other signs to determine whether to keep a baby or not and what kind of future it might have. Other texts mentioning similar traumatic births in association with the birth of a founder ancestor tend to emphasize splitting and cutting. Interestingly, they, like the Chu myth, are pointedly aligned with a non-Zhou cultural identity. The use of medical techniques as an intervention for traumatic births may trace back to the Shang.

> 季繎（連）初降於騩山，氐（抵／至）於空（穴）竆（窮）. 前出於喬（驕）山，宅尻（處）爰波（陂）. 逆上泏水，見盤庚之子，尻（處）于方山，女曰比（妣）隹，秉茲（慈）率相，䍙（麗？離？歷？）冑（迪？遊？）四方. 季繎（連）聞其有聘，從，及之盤（泮），爰生緄伯、遠仲，毓常羊（祥），先尻（處）于京宗.
> 穴酓遟徙於京宗，爰得妣列（瘋？），逆流哉（載）水，厥狀聶耳，乃妻之，生侳叔、麗季. 麗不從行，溃（潰）自脅（脅）出，妣列賓於天，巫戕（咸？）䠱（刻？該？絯？劾？）其脅（脅）以楚，氐（抵／至）今日楚人.

Ji Lian at first descended onto Gui Mountain[21] and then went into a cave 穴竆.[22] Once emerging from Qiao Mountain,[23] he resided at Huanpo, then moving up the Chuan River,[24] he had an audience with Pan Geng's daughter who resided at Fang Mountain. His daughter, named Ancestress Wei (Bird?),[25] had grasped the virtue of compassion. She wandered throughout the Four Regions.[26] Ji Lian heard that she sought marriage, so he pursued her as far as Pan.[27] Eventually, she gave birth to Ying Bo and Yuan Zhong. The delivery was normal and auspicious.[28] At first, they resided in Jingzong (Capital-Main Shrine).

Xue Yin journeyed to Jingzong and eventually got (word of) Ancestress Lie (Break Apart)[29] up the Zai River. She was mature with long delicate ears,[30] so he took her as his wife and she gave birth to Dou Shu and Li Ji. Li did not follow (Shu) (down the birth canal) but came out through a split in her side. Ancestress Lie's (spirit) went to visit Heaven. Shaman Xian (?) cut into (wrapped? confronted the demon in?) her side with thorns,[31] hence the modern term "the People of the Thorns."

In the transmitted tales generally, the youngest and sixth son of the split-side multiple birth was Ji Lian (we note that 6 is a Yin number). The transmitted texts of the birth of the Chu identity do not record the birth of the identifier "Chu" but of a lineage name, Mi 羋, a word that may have been a near homonym with the word for "mother" in archaic Chinese (see chart 5).³² The *Da Dai Liji* adds a few details regarding the mother of Ji Lian in the account preserved in the chapter "Dixi" 帝繫:

陸終氏娶于鬼方氏, 鬼方氏之妹謂之女隤, 氏產六子; 孕而不粥, 三年, 啟其左脅, 六人出焉. 其一曰樊, 是為昆吾; 其二曰惠連, 是為參胡; 其三曰籛, 是為彭祖; 其四曰萊言, 是為云鄶人; 其五曰安, 是為曹姓. 其六曰季連, 是為羋姓.
Chief Lu Zhong took a wife from the chief of the Guifang, a maid called Nü Tui. She produced six children. When she was pregnant, she did not give birth until after three years when her left side split open and six people emerged. The first was named Fan, constituting the Kunwu (people); the second was named Hui Lian, constituting the Canhu; the third was Jian, constituting the Pengzu; the fourth was Laiyan, constituting the Yunkuai people; the fifth was An, constituting the Cao lineage; **the sixth was called Ji Lian, constituting the Mi lineage name.**

In this account, we learn that the wife of Lu Zhong was unable to give birth for three years until finally six children burst out of her left side. The youngest, Ji Lian, was the founder of the Mi lineage.

We find a similar account in the *Shiben* 世本 but with some details similar to those found in the *Shiji*. The *Shiben* account is basically similar to that in the *Da Dai Liji* but with different graphs used for some names, suggesting diverse paths of transmission for the tale.³³

陸終娶于鬼方氏之妹, 謂之女嬇. 是生六子, 孕而不育. 三年, 啟其左脅, 三人出焉, 破其右脅, 三人出焉. 其一曰樊, 是為昆吾. 二曰惠連, 是為參胡. 三曰籛鏗, 是為彭祖. 四曰求言, 是為會人. 其五曰安, 是為曹姓. 六曰季連, 是為羋姓. 昆吾者, 衛是也. 參胡者, 韓是也. 彭祖者, 彭城是也. 會人者, 鄭是也. 曹姓者, 邾是也. 季連者, 楚是也.
Lu Zhong took as wife a maid of the chief of the Guifang, calling her Nü Kui. She gave birth to six children. She was pregnant but did not give birth until after three years, then three burst out of her left side and three burst out of her right side. The first one of those was called Fan, constituting the Kunwu; the second was Huilian, constituting the Canhu; the third was Jian Jian, constituting the Pengzu; the fourth was Qiuyan,

constituting the Hui people; the fifth was An, constituting the Cao lineage; **the sixth child was Ji Lian, constituting the Mi lineage.** The Kunwu are of Wei; the Canhu are of Han; the Pengzu are of Pengcheng; the Hui people are of Kuai; the Cao lineage are of Zhu; **those of Ji Lian are of Chu.**

The origin of the Chu identifier "Thorn" is not explained as in the *Chu ju*, but the name does indicate Ji Lian's offspring. The emphasis on a troublesome birth recalls the *Chu ju* but with the fundamental difference that all the children came out of the woman's sides and not just the last one, the Chu founder.

The "Liu Guo" 六國 chapter of the *Fengsu tongyi* 風俗通義 has a similar account (parts of which can be found as in the "Chu shijia" chapter of the *Shiji*):[34]

> 楚之先出自帝顓頊, 其裔孫曰陸終, 娶于鬼方氏, 是謂女潰. 蓋孕而三年不育, 啟其左脅, 三人出焉, 啟其右脅, 三人又出焉. **其六曰季連, 是為羋.** 其後有鬻熊子為文王師. 成王舉文、武勤勞, 而封熊繹於楚, 食子男之采, 其十世稱王.
>
> The ancestors of Chu came from god-king Zhuanxu and among his descendants was **Lu Zhong, who took a wife from the chief of the Guifang, named Nü Kui.** When she became pregnant, she went three years without producing, until her left side split open and three people came out and her right side split open and three more people came out. **The sixth of them was Ji Lian, who constituted the Mi.** His descendants included the children of **Yu Xiong,** who was a teacher for King Wen (of Zhou). King Cheng promoted the officers who worked diligently for Wen and Wu and gave Xiong Yi a land grant in Chu, providing a salary of *zinan* status, and for ten generations they used the title "king."

This account, like all those examined earlier, emphasizes a three-year pregnancy. Three-year pregnancies appear in other non-Zhou founder birthing myths as well, such as the traumatic births of the founders of the Xia and Shang dynasties, Sage-Kings Yu 禹 and Xie 契. Such split-side tales were so widespread that they persisted into later times. For example, the Eastern Jin author Gan Bao's 干寶 (d. 336) verification of this strange style of birth is cited by the Southern dynasties scholar, Pei Yin 裴駰 (fl. 438) in his commentary, the *Shiji jijie* 史記集解:[35]

先儒學士多疑此事 . . . 然按六子之世，子孫有國，升降六代，數千年間，迭至霸王，天將興之，必有尤物乎？若夫前志所傳，修己背坼而生禹，簡狄胸剖而生契，歷代久遠，莫足相証. 近魏黃初五年，汝南屈雍妻王氏生男兒從右胳下水腹上出，而平和自若，數月創合，母子無恙，斯蓋近事之信也. 以今況古，固知注記者之不妄也.

Early Ru scholars were all skeptical about this . . . with regard to the generations of the six sons whose descendants all had states, they rose and fell for a thousand years, alternating in their roles as hegemonic kings supported by Heaven, must they be prodigies? So much time has passed since the earlier accounts of Yu's birth out of a split in Xiuji (his mother's) back and Xie's birth out of a break in Jiandi's (his mother's) chest that it is impossible now to verify. Recently, however, early in the fifth year of the Wei Huang (224) in Runan, Quyong, a married woman gave birth to a boy through her left armpit, above her abdomen. It came out peacefully and after several months the opening resealed. The mother was unharmed. This is a recent reliable account. So, if it can happen now, it could certainly happen in antiquity. So, we can understand that the commentators were not simply being irresponsible.

Gan Bao, the author of the famous stories of oddities, the *Shoushenji* 搜神记, was a collector of tales. He noted that earlier Ru scholars dismissed the *Shiji* and other accounts of Lu Zhong's split-side birthing. They figured that it was a Chu peoples' effort to self-aggrandize their birthright in order to takeover hegemony of the Central Plains (following the famous *Zuozhuan* account of the Chu request for the sacred Nine Caldrons of Zhou). After hearing about the experience of the Wei lady, however, Gan Bao suggested that the ancient account was indeed true. One difference between the Wei account of the traumatic birth and most of the earlier accounts is focus on the effect on the mother (she survived the ordeal) rather than using it as proof of divine origin.[36] Among the earlier versions, only the *Chu ju* account refers to the effect of the birth on the mother, the manipulation of her body by a shaman, and, finally, her "visit to Heaven."

In the birth tales of the Chu people in the *Shiji*, the *Chu ju*, and later texts, the signature event is of the body of the progenitor or of his female partner splitting open. In other versions of this birthing style with different divine founder kings, such as Sage-King Yu, the body was sometimes replaced with a stone or even a fish, thus further emphasizing the magical nature of the birth.[37] In any case, the child becomes the new founding ancestor of the ruling lineage associated with a new dynasty, one that metaphorically split off from the trunk lineage and from the past. The Chu writer's application of this tale to the Chu lineage actually supports the early scholars' accusation that the Chu were self-aggrandizing, expecting to be the ones who would create a new dynasty and empire (instead of the Qin as actually resulted).

Unlike Gan's account of the Wei lady's experience of the split-side birth, in most cases of the tale, as in the *Chu ju*, the birth of the *name* of the founder, lineage, or polity is more important than the health of people involved, the mother, or even the child/progenitor itself. The Chu people derived their name "Thorny" (*chu* 楚) from the shamanist medical practice of using thorns in dealing with the split-side birth.[38]

As we have seen, one clue to the antiquity or, at least the multiplicity, of different versions of the origins tales is in the overlapping use of and variation in the names of the ancestors. In the genealogies of the Chu house preserved in the *Chu ju*, the *Shiji*, and the *Da Dai Liji* we saw many variations on the names, some that may have been in fact birth mothers but tradition treated them like fathers. We saw this in the case of Ji Lian's offspring named Fu Ju 附沮 (which in fact was written Fu Zu 付祖 for Shizu ren 什祖人 in various texts).[39] In the following, we will summarize the relationships in the Chu genealogical texts. Since all claim that the Chu identity began with Ji Lian, so sections beginning with Ji Lian are in bold. The use of ellipses shows where the texts suggest that more than one generation has passed:

Chu ju: **Ji Lian (with Pangeng's daughter, Ancestress Wei)** ⇨
  Cheng Bo + Yuan Zhong
  Xue Yin (with Ancestress Lie) ⇨ **Shu Shu + Li Li (Chu)**

Shiji ("Chu shijia"): Huangdi ⇨ Changyi ⇨ Di Zhuanxu, Gaoyang ⇨
  Cheng ⇨ Juanzhang (= Lao Tong)[40] ⇨ Chong Li + Wuhui (Zhu Rong); Wu Hui ⇨ Lu Zhong ⇨ Kun Wu + Can Hu +Pengzu + Hui *ren* + Cao *xing* + **Ji Lian (= Mi *xing* = Chu);**
    Ji Lian ⇨ **Xue Xiong** ⇨ **Zhongwei** ⇨ **. . . Yu Xiong** ⇨
    Xiong Li ⇨ **Xiong Kuang** ⇨ **(Chu Man) Xiong Yi**

Da Dai Liji ("Di xi," parts very similar to "Wudi benji" in the *Shiji*):
Huangdi (with Daughter of Xiling, Leizu) ⇨ Qingyang + Changyi; Changyi (with Daughter of the Shu Shan Shi, Chang Pu) ⇨ Zhuanxu ⇨ Qiong Chan + Kun + Lao Tong (mother was runaway daughter of the Zhen shi, Nü Lu); Lao Tong (with Daughter of the Jieshui shi, Gao Gua) ⇨ Chong Li + Wu Hui; Wu Hui ⇨ Lu Zhong (with maid of Guifang shi, Nü Kui) ⇨ Fan (Kun Wu) + Hui Lian (Can Hu) + Jian (Pengzu) + Lai Yan (Kuai *ren*) + An (Cao *xing*) + **Ji Lian (Mi *xing*)**;
Ji Lian ⇨ Shenzu *ren* ⇨ Nei Xiong (=Xue Xiong)[41] . . .

Fengsu Tongyi ("Liu Guo"): Di Zhuanxu . . . Lu Zhong (married Nüzi of the Guifang shi) ⇨ (last of six) **Ji Lian (Mi)** . . . Yu Xiong Zi . . . Xiong Yi

Gender-Bending

An investigation of the multiplicity of ancestral names attributed to the Chu mythical lineage along with a comparison of the ancient pronunciations of the names listed in chart 5 allows us to make the following observations: first, Wu Hui and Fu Ju fall in the female category. Wu Hui's name was very close to the pronunciations of the names for Lu Zhong's wife. Note, too, that the clan name given to the Chu people in the transmitted texts, Mi 羋 (and perhaps Fuxi? Note the correspondence of the second syllable with names in the female list), must also by the same logic belong in the female category. Fu Ju's name is less obvious, but the ending syllable places it a category of pronunciation combining aspects of the names of the wives of Huangdi and Changyi. The names of Huangdi and Changdi were near rhymes. The name of Changyi's wife may be simply a feminine form of his name. The names Lao Tong, Zhu Rong, and Lu Zhong are near rhymes. The names Zhu Rong and Yu Yin rhyme if we consider the alternative pronunciation for Rong. A number of the male names have "*-ang" finals, although some begin with velar initials (Huang, Kuang) and some with dentals (Chang minus the prefix, Zhang). Most curious is the occurrence of words that end with a high vowel "*-i" or final "*-it": Li of Chong Li, Ji of Ji Lian and Li Ji, and Xue of Xue Xiong and Xue Yin. In fact, Ji and Xue were near homonyms, both with rounded velar initials (as with some in the female series but with a-j final), forcing us to examine the low back vowel and dental nasal final of Lian ("*-an") (and the Xi of Baoxi's "*-ar," the "*-aj" of Xi of Fuxi is curiously close to one of the readings for Wa of Nüwa) as a possible corruption of the middle or low rounded back vowels (followed by bilabial nasals) of Xiong or Yin ("*-əm, -um"). Or was it a corruption of the male "*-ang" final names? The only other names that end with a dental final ("*-t") are in the female name category. It is possible that the Li of Li Ji and Xiong Li may have been a near rhyme with the Lie of Bi Lie in the female category.

What does such speculation about rhyme, near rhyme, and gender-bending tell us? It tells us that the confusion and profusion of different names for figures representing prehistorical or mythical time periods of Chu lineage history evident in the different accounts may stem from crisscrossing over time of narrative strands in oral tales associated with the origins of certain groups of people. Writers picked those strands that they were most familiar with, perhaps attempting to read fragmented old texts (or bits of old stories), and rearranged them in an order that made sense to them. Some storytellers included birth mothers and others did not.

The Baoshan divination text, also from the fourth-century BCE Chu area, acknowledges three separate groups of ancestral spirits, two of which are linked to legendary kings: one group consisting of the Three Chu Progenitors and another group of five historical kings. The group of three progenitors includes Lao Tong, Zhu Rong, and Yu Yin (= Yu Xiong). The group of historical kings is referred to only as "Jing Kings from Yin Lu up to Wu Wang" 荊王自酓鹿以就武王. We know that the last king referred to was Chu king Wu (r. 740–690 BCE). From the *Chu ju* text, we can see that Lu 鹿 was probably a shortened version of Li 麗, son of Xue Yin 穴酓.⁴² Although the *Chu ju* does not make clear the relationship between the descended spirit Ji Lian and Ancestress Lie's male partner Xue Yin, the more complete *Shiji* genealogy clearly lists Xue Xiong (assumed to be Xue Yin) as the offspring of Ji Lian. In transmitted texts, Xue Xiong and Yu Xiong both had sons named Li, either called Li Ji 麗季 (*rˤə-s-C.rəʔ) or Xiong Li 熊麗 (*C.ɢʷəm-C.rəʔ).⁴³ The ubiquity of the name Li and the parallels between father and son figures hint at the later elaboration of earlier tales that were imperfectly remembered or transmitted—a metaphorical twinning of an original progenitor myth. The connections between these figures in transmitted and newly discovered texts also allow us to link the two groups of progenitors listed separately in the Baoshan text, yet preserve the distinction that Li was the acknowledged progenitor of the Chu identity.

Chart 5. Chu ancestral names

Male

♦Huangdi 黃帝	*[ɢ]ʷˤaŋ-tˤek-s	
♦Changyi 昌意	*mə-tʰaŋ-ʔ(r)ək-s	
♦Gaoyang 高陽	*Cə.[k]ˤaw-laŋ	
Zhuanxu 顓頊	*ton-qʰ(r)ok	
Cheng 稱	*tʰəŋ	
♦Juan Zhang 卷章	*[k](r)o[n]ʔ-taŋ	
■Lao Tong 老童	*C.rˤuʔ-[d]ˤoŋ	
•Chong Li 重黎	*[m]-troŋ-[r]ˤi	
□■Zhu Rong 祝融	*[t]uk-luŋ (lum)	
■Lu Zhong 陸終	*[r]uk-N-t<r>oŋʔ-s	
•Ji Lian 季連	*kʷi[t]-[r]a[n]	
•Xue Xiong 穴熊	*[ɢ]ʷi[t]-C.[ɢ]ʷ(r)əm	
□•Xue Yin 穴僑	*[ɢ]ʷi[t]-q(r)[u]mʔ	
□Yu Xiong 鬻熊	*m-quk-C.[ɢ]ʷ(r)əm	
□Yu Yin 毓僑	*m-quk-q(r)[u]mʔ	
?•Li Ji 麗季	*[r]ˤe-kʷi[t]	
?Xiong Li 熊麗	*C.[ɢ]ʷ(r)əm-[r]ˤe-s	
♦Xiong Kuang 熊狂	*C.[ɢ]ʷ(r)əm-[k-ɢʷ]aŋ	
Xiong Yi 熊繹	*C.[ɢ]ʷ(r)əm-lAk	

Chu 楚 *s.r̥aʔ
Jing 荊 *[k]reŋ

?Fuxi 伏羲 *[b]ək-ŋ̊(r)aj

Pao Xi 庖羲 *[b]ˤruŋ̊(r)aj
Da Xiong Baoxi
 大熊雹戲 *lˤ at-C.[ɢ]ʷ(r)əm-C.[b]ˤruk-(r)ar-s

Nü Tian 女填 *nraʔ-[d]ˤi[n]
Nü Huang 女皇 *nraʔ-[ɢ]ʷˤaŋ

Female

Liezu 累祖 *[r]oj- [ts]ˤaʔ
 纍祖 *[r]uj-[ts]ˤaʔ
 雷祖 *C.rˤuj-[ts]ˤaʔ

Changpu 昌僕 *mə-tʰaŋ-[b]ˤok
 昌仆 *mə-tʰaŋ-pʰok-s

♀Wu Hui 吳回 *ŋʷˤa-[ɢ]ʷˤəj

Nü Tui 女隤 *nraʔ-N-rˤuj
Nü Kui 女嬇 *nraʔ-[gʷ]ˤ[ə]j-s
 (kʰˤ ru[t]-s)
 女潰 *nraʔ-[gʷ]ˤ[ə]j-s

Bi Wei 妣隹 *pijʔ-ɢʷij (ɢʷujʔ)
♀Fu Ju 附沮 *N-p(r)oʔ-[dz]aʔ
Bi Lie 妣列 *pijʔ-[r][e]t

♀Mi 羋 *[m-ŋ]e(j)ʔ
 (Mou 牟 *mə, mˤ(r)u)

Mu 母 *məʔ (*mˤoʔ)

Nü Gua/Wo/Wa 女媧 *nraʔ-kʷˤra[j]ʔ (k.rˤoj, kˤrə)

While both sets of genealogies would suggest a temporal linear relationship of human figures, the addition of supernatural aspects allows us to examine some of the imagery as satisfying mythical or imaginary criteria. For example, in some ways the two *Chu ju* figures, Ji Lian ("kʷitran") and Xue Yin ("ɢʷˤit[q]rum?"), were shadows of each other, metaphorical twins. Ji Lian first lived in a cave after descending into the mortal world, and Xue Yin's name is made up of "Cave" (*xue*) and "Drink" (*yin*) or "Bear" (*xiong*). One might speculate that the two figures represented two different legends associated with a single "split" progenitor, one the father of an auspicious birth and the other of a tragic birth. This is complicated by the fact that Yu Xiong ("m-quɢʷrəm," or Yu Yin, "m-qukrum?"), the potential "Birth" deity, seems to be another name for Xue Yin or Xue Xiong. In the *Shiji*, the descendants of Xue Xiong were split between the Central States (Yellow River culture) and the nonassimilated peoples of the Yangzi River valley (e.g., the Manyi). Yu Xiong represented those descendants that lived among the barbarians (although, apparently, his sons served the Zhou court, suggesting that Yu Xiong theoretically lived right around the time when the Zhou conquered the Shang). Hence, the birth of the Chu identity was understood as almost contemporary to the birth of the Zhou state. Historians try to keep the names with the different prefixes, Xue versus Yu, separate, but in fact they became confused, and it seems all represent aspects of a single Chu progenitor.

Whether the Chu prefix Yu can be traced back to the Shang group term for ancestral spirits will probably never be known. In the *Chu ju*, the only link between the Shang and Chu cultures evident in the *Chu ju* is the mythological claim of descent from a Shang princess. The divinely descended Ji Lian of the *Chu ju*, like Lu Zhong (= Zhu Rong) of the transmitted texts, mated with women of the Shang era: Lu Zhong with a young woman of the Gui people (who may have fought with the Shang and Zhou from the north), and Ji Lian with a daughter or granddaughter of the migrant Shang king Pan Geng. Instead of the multiple births of either Lu Zhong or Ji Lian in the transmitted histories, the *Chu ju* documents two births of twins by two separate mothers. Since the birthing of twins in progenitor myths is common worldwide, we look more closely to this metaphor of the Chu identity forming as a result of splitting.

6

The Traumatic Births of Non-Zhou Ancestral Founders

The Chu traumatic birth tale is found in other texts primarily representing regions outside of the Central Plains of the central Yellow River area and dominated by late Zhou culture. The purposeful selection of a princess from the pre-Zhou polity of Shang, one dominating the eastern region, suggests a Chu attempt to link itself to a minority tradition that celebrates a discourse not dominated by Zhou cultural hegemony. It also hints at an unusual celebration of the female ancestor, who like a goddess could come to earth or return to heaven as needed. Most striking is the use of the tale of a "split-side" (*xie sheng* 脅生) birth[1] that has been associated in other texts with the births of pre-Zhou dynastic founders of the Xia and Shang. The Han and later texts featuring the "split-side" birthing tales of founders suggest a southeastern story cycle reflected in its earliest incarnations in late Warring States–period texts, such as the *Chuci* and the *Shanhaijing*, and reproduced in such Han texts as the *Huainanzi* 淮南子, *Chunqiu fanlu* 春秋繁露, *Qianfu lun* 潛夫論, and *Wu Yue chunqiu* 吳越春秋.[2] Although we assume from the script style of the *Chu ju* and from the mere fact of its survival that it had been preserved in a tomb in the Jiangling region of Hubei Province, the later popularity of this style of birthing tale in the eastern Yangzi River valley region suggests that either the Chu helped to spread it eastward or that the Chu had absorbed parts of the tale from the eastern regions in the first place. In any case, by the end of the Han period, the tale was well known even in the western regions. It even appears in the writings of a famous physician from Gansu, Huangfu Mi 皇甫謐 (215–282), who had been schooled in the Zhou culturally dominated Confucian classics.

The split-side birth, a characteristic of Chu identity, is purposefully contrasted with the smooth birth of twins by the Shang princess. But it also contrasts with the well-known legend of an auspicious and pain-free birth of the Zhou ancestor Hou Ji by Jiang Yuan. The ode "Birth of the People" ("Shengmin"), mentioned in chapter 2, describes the divine conception and auspicious birth of the agricultural deity, Hou Ji, whom Han editors subsequently documented as the founding ancestor of the Zhou people.[3] In Western Zhou inscriptions, Hou Ji was worshipped as an earth god, opposite the sky god, Shangdi.[4] In the *Book of Odes*, Shangdi impregnates the Zhou ancestress Jiang Yuan while she performed a shamanistic fertility ritual. In this tale, only the father was of divine origins, not the female ancestor. The name Jiang Yuan 姜嫄 combines the lineage name of Jiang 姜, the surname typically carried by Zhou royal brides, with a personal name phonetically homophonous with the word "origin" (*yuan* 原) (and the words for enclosure and spring discussed in terms of the Shang word for "to give birth" in chapter 1). The record of Jiang Yuan's birthing experience is important to our study, because the *Chu ju* seems to consciously make a distinction between smooth auspicious births and those that involved splitting apart and harm. Jiang Yuan did not require a midwife but was guided and protected by Shangdi. Women without the divine aid of this Zhou-approved god were in danger of traumatic birthing experiences and perhaps even death. Her auspicious birthing experience is described in the ode as follows:

誕彌厥月、先生如達 (祥?)、不坼不副、無菑無害.
以赫厥靈、上帝不 (丕?) 寧、不 (丕?) 康禋祀、居然生子.
As those months extended and drew near, her first birth was like a lamb (auspicious? 祥),[5] no tearing, no splitting, no injury, no harm.
Such a magnificent spirit as Shangdi, so tranquil and content with the pure wine and annual sacrifices; so, too, was the birth of the child.

The fact that this birthing account emphasizes the lack of splitting and tearing suggests a purposeful contrast with contemporaneous but non-surviving versions of split-style birthing myths. As we shall see, these included the Shang origin birth myth mentioned earlier. This suggests that the split-side-style birthing legends were as old as this Zhou song, which was possibly not as ancient as tradition claims—the early Western Zhou period (mid-eleventh to mid-tenth centuries BCE), presumably the same time period as Xue Yin (or Yu Xiong)—but certainly earlier than the fourth century BCE.[6] Hence, we might guess that tales of split-side births, if not some aspect of the phenomenon itself, trace back even further in history than the *Chu ju*.

In a speculative reach back into time, we might consider the sophisticated nature of late Shang society, which perhaps, like the Egyptians and Romans, may actually have employed a type of cesarean section birth that was not understood by the cruder western tribes that constituted the early Zhou people. We note that the Zhou word for the Shang people, Yin 殷, consisted of a graphical depiction of a hand with an implement pointed at a pregnant belly (see chart 6). In later myth, one of the sins attributed to the last Shang kings was cutting open pregnant women (*ti yunfu* 剔孕婦) and other surgical operations, such as cutting open Prince Bigan's chest to view his heart (*pou Bigan xin* 剖比干心).[7] The Zhou interpreted these operations upon the human body as abominations rather than as surgical procedures. Scholar Liu Xinfang notes that such surgeries were certainly known by the Three Kingdoms period and the cesarean procedure may have been historically a technique of last resort to save an heir.[8]

Chart 6. Images of technical intervention in pregnancy

Shang graph for *yin* 殷 (*ʔər), a medical technique

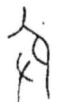 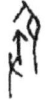

Western Zhou graphs for Yin, a name for the Shang

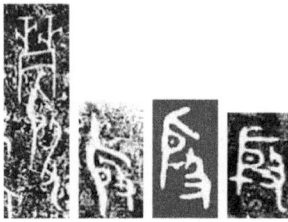

The word *yin* is very rare in the oracle bones. By the late Shang and up through the Zhou periods it was used in personal names as well as the Zhou name for the Shang polity. The examples in chart 6 are found on bronze inscriptions dating from left to right, late Shang (a personal name with a Li 麗 or Lu 鹿 element added), and early, middle, and late Western Zhou (all referring to the Shang polity or people).[9] Many other examples show shortened or more ornate variations (some others also with a "roof" element 宀) that explain the eventual transcription into the more modern 殷 (*ʔər) instead of the earlier more graphic depiction of a body 身 and a hand holding an implement. The graph of the hand holding the implement could have also been transcribed as *yin* 尹 (*m-qurʔ) (instead of 攴), a type of technical officer or manager (or "to manage, govern" when used as a verb).

In the oracle bones, the word *yin* was used as a verb, referring possibly to some means of healing illness (*ji* 疾). It is possible that the core word was more related to the word *yin* (尹 "technician") element rather than the "body" element. The mark indicating something inside the belly seems to distinguish the graph as a pregnant body. Yu Xingwu 于省吾 suggested that the mark represented the illness that required curing. Based on Han and later medical texts, he thought that the method might have been a kind of massage.[10] In fact, illness in ancient China was invariably considered the result of malign supernatural influence, and one method described in fourth-century BCE texts for exorcising it was "to attack" (*gong* 攻), presumably threatening the ghost with a sharp object. One example of the verb *yin* was written with two 束 elements, possibly representing "thorns." Unfortunately, the oracle bone records are so cryptic that we cannot discern if the patient was male or female or any further details about the procedure.[11] It is unfortunate that there are no surviving pre-Han medical manuscripts to provide further hints. What remain are numerous tales of the traumatic "split-side" births of non-Zhou progenitors.

The narrative of split-side births was not unknown to the Chu writers. Roughly contemporary versions, although none having directly to do with the birth of the Chu people, are found in the Chu Silk Manuscript, the *Zigao* 子羔 bamboo text, and the *Shanhaijing*. The metaphor of "splitting" for the birth of non-Zhou dynastic founders seems to be a constant. In the *Chu ju*, the mother of the Chu progenitor was named "Break Apart" (Lie), and she physically split apart when the second twin burst out through her rib cage.

The Chu Silk Manuscript has a birth tale also not found in transmitted literature that involves both a father and mother figure, generally understood by scholars to represent the mythical progenitors, Fuxi 伏羲 and Nüwa 女娲. In the manuscript, Fuxi was called Da Xiong Baoxi 大熊雹戲 and Nüwa was called Nü Tian 女填 (or possibly Nü Huang 女皇). As a couple, they are popularly found in Han-period transmitted texts and in tomb art, either in association with bears, dragons, or snakes.[12] Although the silk manuscript is damaged, scholars have been able to decipher that the woman gave birth to four sons, one of whom was Yu and another, Xie (曰古囗大熊雹戲 . . . 乃娶〔夙沙〕囗之子曰女填, 是生子四 . . . 为禹为契).[13] The focus in this text was the role of the four divinities (the other names are unclear) in controlling time, particularly with the progression of the four seasons. They also caused the split of the cosmos into Above and Below. The movement of each founder deity was indicated by the change in seasons. The Creator god was Da Xiong Fuxi. The addition of the Chu title *xiong* "Bear" to Fuxi suggests either that Fuxi was a Chu god or that this manuscript represents a Chu attempt at ownership of this tale. The *Shiben* claims that Huangdi was responsible for a Xiong lineage (a Han appropriation of Chu history).

The graph for Xiong was actually written with a "Big" (*da* 大) semantic element on top as a single graph. We suspect then that perhaps 大 was confused with 穴 and that Xue Xiong and Fuxi, two creators from different story cycles, were joined in this manuscript. This supports Qiu Xigui's idea that Yu Xiong/Yu Yin/Xue Yin/Da Xiong may have been the same creator god as Taiyi, because both are credited with the birth of the cosmos and time.[14] As we saw earlier, Taiyi took shape (or stored his/her energy) inside water, much as a spring does inside its earth enclosure. The Chu Silk Manuscript attributes the movement from environmental chaos to order—commonly associated with Sage-King Yu—instead of a divine Chu founder and his descendants. In a bamboo text stored in the Shanghai Museum, the *Rongchengshi* 容成氏, Yu was associated with a bear (or a tortoise, Nai?) written the same as the Chu title 熊.[15] Whether the Chu mythmakers simply appropriated earlier Yu (the sage and founder of Xia) and Fuxi/Nüwa legends for their own political purposes or originally felt some deeper ancestral link between them and Chu is difficult to determine at this time.

The Warring States text, the *Zigao*, discussed earlier in the section on fertility prayers in chapter 2, was also from the Chu region. It describes the births of Sage-King Yu and Xie.[16] It distinctly refers to the magical nature of their births, placing the narrative of the Chu founder's birth in the same myth cycle as other non-Zhou founders. It also incorporates features of the Gaomei ritual as well. The *Zigao* describes the three births of dynastic founders, Yu of Xia, Xie (also meaning "split") of Shang, and Hou Ji of Zhou. Unlike the auspicious birth of Hou Ji as described previously, the births of Yu and Xie both involved split-side births (as well as likely forays to Gaomei–like sites).[17]

[禹之母，有莘氏之]女也，觀薏苡而得之，懷三年而劃于背而生，生而能言，是禹也。
契之母，有娀氏之女也。游于陽台之上，有燕銜卵而措諸其前，取而吞之，娠三年而劃于膺，生乃呼曰"金（欽），"是契也。

Yu's mother was a girl of the Xins. When she noticed Job's Tears, she picked some. After a three-year pregnancy, her back split open and Yu was born. The one born who could already talk was Yu.

Xie's mother was a girl of the Rongs. When she traveled to the top of Yangtai (mountain or a high platform), there appeared a swallow with an egg in its beak, which he placed in front of her. She took it and swallowed it. After a three-year pregnancy, her chest split open. The one born who shouted out "Act Respectfully!" was Xie.

The context in the *Zigao* concerns the divine births of three divine founder kings, Yu (Xia), Xie (Shang), and Hou Ji (Zhou). All were magically conceived (eating Job's Tears or an egg in the case of Yu and Xie, stepping on a toe print or footprint in the case of Hou Ji), but only Yu and Xie's births involved three years of pregnancy and a violent birth, in this case, "splitting open" the back or chest. It is perhaps no coincidence that the word *xie* 契, the name of the Shang progenitor, could also mean "split" or "to cut with a knife." This myth cycle reinforces the interpretation that the shaman Xian used the thorn to poke or cut rather than to sew.

In the transmitted textual tradition, specifically from the late Warring States and Han periods, Yu was invariably the product of a split-side birth, often after a three-year gestation, but not always from an identifiable female or mother. For example, in the *Shanhaijing* and *Chuci*, Yu (also known as "Yellow Dragon") was born from his evil father Gun's 鯀 belly (probably also a water creature) (Gun fu sheng Yu 鯀腹

生禹).¹⁸ The *Shanhaijing* refers to the splitting of Gun's dead body. The corpse had miraculously not rotted even after three years (notably the same number of years Lu Zhong's wife was pregnant).¹⁹ Someone cut open the body with "a blade from Wu" (a southeastern coastal state legendary for casting multi-alloyed swords) causing the body to come alive as Yellow Dragon.

Some versions of the tale are associated with the *Guizang* 歸藏 divination manual by later scholars, such as by Guo Pu 郭璞 (276–324). One example of a bit of tale involving the birth of the cosmos in an excavated version of the divination manual was discussed earlier. The transmitted version is preserved as quotes in other texts. The story thread of Yu emerging from Gun's body after three years is preserved in the "Hainei jing" 海內經 chapter of the *Shanhaijing*.

Quoting the "Kaishi" 啟筮 hexagram of the *Guizang*:²⁰

鯀死, 三歲不腐. 剖之以吳刀, 化為黃龍.
After Gun died, his body did not rot for three years. When cut open with a Wu blade, it transformed into a Yellow Dragon.

From the *Guizang* "Qishi" 啓筮 hexagram:²¹

鯀殛死, 三歲不腐, 副之以吳刀, 是用出禹.
Gun was put to death but, after three years, his body had not rotted. It was cut open with a Wu knife to let Yu out.

A thread of the tale is reflected in "Tianwen" 天問 of the *Chuci*:²²

順欲成功, 帝何刑焉?
永遏在羽山, 夫何三年不施 (弛)?
伯禹愎 (腹) 鯀, 夫何以變化?
"If Di's will was accomplished, why did he punish him (Gun)? Long he lay cast off at Feather Mountain; why for three whole years did he not rot? When Lord Yu came forth from Gun's belly, how was he transformed?"

If we replace the symbolism of the evil father Gun with that of the unfortunate mother, then we can see a parallel with the birth of the Chu progenitor from the punished and sliced body. The body of Gun after three years—the same time period prescribed for formal mourning of high-status males—transforms into a dragon, the same form as the transformed body of Lady Dai of the Mawangdui tomb depicted in her funeral painting (and the depictions of the intertwined snake/dragon bodies of Fuxi and Nüwa found outside Han tomb gates).²³ Han texts provide varying accounts. In the *Huainanzi*, "Yu was born from a stone" (*Yu sheng yu shi* 禹生于石), a fact that links him to the myth of Nüwa's creation of the cosmos according to Mark E. Lewis.²⁴ It also links Yu to later mythical cycles of spiritual beings, such as Sun Wukong, the Monkey King, who was born of stone and wielded the staff of the Great Sage Yu in *Journey to the West* and to the protagonist "Precious Jade" (Baoyu) of *Dream of the Red Chamber*.²⁵ In the *Chunqiu fanlu*, "Yu was born out of the back" (*Yu sheng fa yu bei* 禹生發于背), a tale suggesting a birth with unfortunate consequences for the mother and a link to the earlier *Zigao* version. The *Lunheng*, as in the *Zigao*, contrasts Yu's birth with that of Hou Ji: "Yu and Xie had abnormal births; they opened their mothers' backs and came out. Hou Ji had a smooth birth, no tearing or cutting" 禹契逆生, 闓母背而出. 后稷順生, 不坼不副.²⁶

In some versions of the tale of Yu's birth, not only were female birth mothers recognized, but they are also given names as we saw in the *Chu ju* and in some Han versions of progenitors. Gao You 高誘 (fl. 205–212) in a commentary on Yu's birth from a stone in the *Huainanzi* claimed, "When Yu's mother, Xiuji ("Self-cultivated"), felt the imminent birth of Yu, her chest split open and out he emerged" (*Yu mu Xiuji, gan ersheng Yu, che xiong er chu* 禹母修己, 感而生禹, 拆胸而出).²⁷ In the *Wu Yue Chunqiu*, this "split-side" style of birth was described as "splitting open the sides (or ribs)" (*pou xie* 剖脅). The description of Yu's birth in the *Wu Yue Chunqiu* included both name and pedigree for his mother:²⁸

> 鯀娶於有莘氏之女, 名曰女嬉. 年壯未孳, 嬉于砥山, 得薏苡而吞之, 意若為人所感, 因而妊孕, 剖脅而產高密.
> Gun took a woman of the Xin tribe as a wife; her name was Nü Xi. She was mature but had not yet bred. Xi played around on Whetstone Mountain, getting Job's Tears and swallowing them down. She felt as if the making of a person was intended, so she became pregnant and produced Gao Mi through a split in her side.

In this case, pregnancy involved going to a mountain, similar to the *Chu ju* tales, but also swallowing magical seed. Yu, called Gao Mi 高密 in this version, typically came out of a split in her side. The version told by Huangfu Mi in his *Diwang shiji* 帝王世紀 included the father, the mother with pedigree, mountains, and a few new details:[29]

鯀納有莘氏女, 曰志, 是為修己. 上山行, 見流星貫昴, 夢接意感, 又吞神珠薏苡(薏苡), 胸坼而生禹于石紐.

Gun ... brought in a girl of the You Xin tribe called Zhi ("Intention"). This was Xiuji ("Self-cultivated"). While traveling up in the mountains, she saw a falling star piercing the Mao region (of the sky). Then in a dream, she received and felt it, so upon swallowing a divine pearl and Job's Tears, her chest split open and she gave birth to Yu at Stone Knob.

The additional features include the divine nature of the pregnancy but also the name of the place of birth. Her pregnancy resulted from ingesting the same magical seeds as well as a divine pearl, but perhaps even more critical was the supernatural influence from a falling star. Additionally, we learn that instead of birth from a stone, Yu was born at a place called "Stone Knob." In the "Wu de zhi" 五德志 chapter of the *Qianfu lun*, the name Xiu Ji is written differently and not clearly identified as a woman, but only as a "descendant." But, similarly, she (or he?) feels the intended birth after seeing a falling star and produces the Bai Di 白帝 ("White Deity"), Wen Ming, the Great Yu 後嗣脩紀, 見流星, 意感生白帝文命戎禹.[30] In this version, we also see the longer *Wu Yue Chunqiu* statement *yi ruo wei ren suo gan* 意若為人所感 shortened to simply *yigan* 意感. What part of the sky the falling star came from is not specified, and the birth results in one of the Deities of the Five Agents (*wuxing*) who seems to be confused with Yu. Clearly, a tale is being retold over time, adding and subtracting well-worn words to fit the occasion.

Variations of the theme included other characters. We even see hints of it in the tale of the beginning of the Manyi people south of the Yangzi River region (Changsha, specifically) told in the chapter "Nan Man Xinan Yi liezhuan" 南蠻西南夷列傳 of the *Hou Han shu*. A few details might even be considered curiously reminiscent of the *Chu ju* and other later versions. This is the tale of a younger daughter of Di Ku, the chief of the Gao Xin people 高辛氏. She married the dog Pan Hu 槃瓠 after he met Di's challenge to capture an enemy general. Pan Hu carried his wife up into the Southern Mountains where they lived in a stone room 石室 in a region far from people. After three years, she had twelve children, six boys and six girls who interbred after the death of their father (the dog). The mother finally returned to meet with Bai Di (the White Deity = Di Ku), who authorized a mountainous land called Guangze 廣澤 as their homeland where they became known as the Manyi.[31]

It seems that the tale of the origins of the southern peoples share important features with birth narratives of the Xia, Shang, and Chu progenitors. The *Shiji* suggests that the earliest Chu polity was set among the Manyi. Similarities include the births taking place in the mountains, involving three years and multiples of children. The women came from people named Xin. In the *Chu ju*, Ji Lian first lived in a cave, whereas in the *Hou Han shu* version, Pan Hu and his wife lived in a "stone room." In the *Chu ju* one of the ancestor's names was Pan Geng 盤庚 (ca. 1300 BCE), an itinerant Shang king who was the first to split off his people and settle at Yinxu in Anyang,[32] whereas in the *Hou Han shu* it was Pan Hu, a dog who ran off into the uninhabited hills. In the Huangfu Mi version, Yu's birth occurred at "Stone Knob" (Shiniu 石紐). Yang Xiong 揚雄 (53 BCE–18 CE) claimed that Stone Knob was in Guangrou District in the mountains around the Wen River in Sichuan 汶山廣柔縣.[33] Curiously, the mountainous homeland of the Manyi people in the *Hou Han shu* was named Guangze 廣澤, although the places historically connected with these two early names were nowhere near each other.

In contemporaneous tales of split-side births, we also find a curious mixing up of the vocabulary and verbs with nouns that suggest an old tale with more modern variants. In these stories, instead of the verb "to split" *kui* 潰 (gʷˤəj-s) as found in the *Chu ju*, the mothers' names are Tui, Kui, or Gui, written variously as 隤, 嬇, or 鬼 (k-ʔuj?), but the verb "to split" was written as *qi* 啟 (kʰˤijʔ). The names and the verbs used were all very close in pronunciation as, in fact, was the name of the mountain Ji Lian descended to in the *Chu ju* (畏 ʔuj-s) and his wife's name (隹 gʷij). Such correlations suggest that variants of the myths were orally transmitted with key words replaced or recontextualized as necessary. It also suggests that by the time of the *Chu ju*, the original tale—if there was one—was lost and had to be recreated.

In any case, it is clear that the tales involving split-side-style births can be traced to at least the late Warring States period. Qiu Xigui noted that the tale of the Great Sage Yu being born from Gun's belly mentioned in the *Shanhaijing* and in the "Tianwen" in the *Chuci* most likely had earlier regional origins and represented a local tradition.[34] In the transmission of split-side birth tales, the version with Gun seems to have been replaced in popularity with the versions involving women. Symbols of fertility and reproduction, such as the woman consuming a pearl, seed, or egg, became important details during the Han period. The tale of the parallel "abnormal births" (*nisheng* 逆生) of both Yu and Xie from their mothers' backs in the Warring States–period *Zigao* persisted as a key element in later versions of the tale, such as in Wang Chong's 王充 (27–100? CE) chapter of oddities, the "Qiguai pian" 奇怪篇, in the *Lunheng* 論衡, and even later in the writings of Eastern Jin–period author Gan Bao. The tales of auspicious births mentioned earlier that purposely contrast the smoothness of birth (as in Jiang Yuan's of Hou Ji) suggests that both types of birthing tales had ancient origins.

The two-sided style of the female birthing experience of the Chu people reflects the hybrid nature of Chu culture in the late Warring States period—strong currents of Zhou influence overlaid older influences, some of which were shared with the late-Shang Anyang culture. The imagery of splitting in China is ancient. It is reflected in the ritual decor on bronze vessels, divination and other religious practices, and, now, even in this chronicle of the history of "dwellings" (*ju*) of the Chu leaders. The primitive style of the basic chronicle-style "X settled at Y place" and genealogical-style "A begat (or "fathered") B" records is common in Han histories and is found to some degree in the earlier *Chunqiu*. In this sense, the Chu text fits neatly into the literary milieu of Yellow River culture. On the other hand, we know that by the late Warring States period the state of Chu had already moved from the west to the east, dominated the Huai River 淮河 valley, and connected cultures all along the Yangzi River.

The reflection of the split nature of Chu identity in the *Chu ju* is what distinguishes it from the later Han-period accounts. First, it right off the bat claims heritage to a Shang king famous for splitting off his branch of the Shang people and migrating with them to the southern side of the Yellow River. Second, it records two contrasting female birthing experiences, both critical to the birth and naming of the Chu identity as represented by the name "Thorny." The two births symbolize the split identity in a multilayered pattern, again an artistic trait of Warring States Chu art that can be traced back to the so-called "mask" or split-image decor in Shang art.[35]

The first birth, the birth of twin sons to Ji Lian and their Shang mother, Ancestress Wei, was smooth and auspicious, but the second birth of twins to Xue Yin and Ancestress Lie (from the Zai River region) resulted in a death and a birth: the death of the mother and the birth of Chu ancestor Li Ji. The woman who was "split open" in the Han accounts was named Gui or Kui. These graphs represented homophones for the verb *kui* used in the *Chu ju* to describe the traumatic split-open birth (潰 *gʷˤəj-s). In the *Chu ju*, the mother's name, Ancestress Lie 列 (pronounced *ret), also meant to "break apart."[36] The symbolic splitting off is replicated in the birth of twins and the fact that it was the second twin that caused the death of the mother.

Tales of twins in which one child has a normal birth and the other child's is troublesome are common in many other parts of the ancient world. One example from the Iroquois people is striking. The "maize mother" represents a goddess descended from Heaven to the Earth. She became pregnant with a "good" and "bad" twin by having sharp and blunt arrows pressed against her body. The good child came out the natural way, but the bad child came out of a split in the side of her body, causing her to die and for maize to rise through her corpse. This symbolized the beginning of Earth.[37] In the *Chu ju*, it was the second child, Li Ji ("rekʷit"), who refused to follow (*bu cong xing* 不從行) the first good child, causing his mother's body to split. It was the thorns used in the birth process that symbolized the beginning of the Chu people. Thorns, like arrows in ancient Chinese texts, may have had an exorcist or magical function.

In summary, unique, or potentially non-Zhou cultural aspects, of the *Chu ju* tale include:

1. Ji Lian was not born of a split-side birth but descended like a god down to a mountain.

2. His own sons' births were smooth, conforming to Zhou-style tales but contrasting with the subsequent birth of twins for his doppelganger, Xue Yin.

3. The birth of the name for the Chu people follows the Xia/Shang origin-mythic style of a split-side birth but with added details relevant to the birth.

Although this splitting of Chu tradition from the Zhou and of the body of the mother symbolized in the two types of births and by Ancestress Lie were clearly important symbolic transitions in the generation of the Chu people, if this were the only genealogical narrative in existence for the Chu, we would know very little about the early male lineage. This vagueness is exacerbated by the double-gendered nature implicated by the names for Xue Yin, presumably Ancestress Lie's mate.

The birth tales of dynastic progenitors contrast the Zhou with the Xia, Shang, and Chu traditions. The *Chu ju* itself proclaims a Shang connection through an ancestress, and while there are tantalizing cultural threads to a Shang past, it is impossible to verify. We know from the oracle bones discovered in Shaanxi in a building dated to the first half of the early Western Zhou period that people by the name of Chu existed. By the middle Western Zhou period, bronze inscriptions document military expeditions to the south to attack the Chu Jing peoples 楚荊. In fact, archaeologists trace the rise and fall of numerous cultures in the middle and lower Yangzi River valley since the early Neolithic period. The Shang seemed to have colonial links to the middle Yangzi through their metal-producing settlement at modern Panlongcheng 盤龍城. The Western Zhou and Yangzi cultures communicated through Han River 漢水 peoples who may have been "Chu" and/or "Jing." During the Spring and Autumn period and up through the Warring States period, the state better known as Chu, based in the Han River valley and at Jiangling on the Yangzi, expanded eastward and northward. Texts found in Chu tombs confirm that the educated elite of the Chu state participated in the general cultural milieu of the early Chinese civilization, which included the older and more sophisticated Yellow River valley cultures.[38] By the time of the late Warring States period and the writing of the *Chu ju*, the political elite of Chu had moved eastward toward the coast to escape the invading Qin.

No other text besides the *Chu ju* makes such specific claims for a connection to the Shang. This cultural heritage is claimed through the mother not the father. Ji Lian went up the Chuan River to visit with a "child" 子 of Pan Geng, a legendary Shang king (逆上洲水, 見盤庚之子), a familiar trope in genealogical tales of the Han period. By the late Warring States period, Pan Geng was a familiar legend. He was famous for forcing the Shang people to migrate from place to place before settling, just like the twenty-three Chu rulers chronicled in the *Chu ju*. He was also credited with naming the people as Yin (even though the name Yin first appears in Zhou inscriptions). Hence, he was not only an ancestor but a noble historical model as well. There may be a political motivation in adopting this genealogy, as Gan Bao earlier questioned.

Some scholars locate the prehistoric Chu realm of influence as stretching from the Dan River area in northern Henan as far north as Lantian 藍田 in Shaanxi. They may have come in contact with the

Shang when pushing eastward in the boundary region between the Jing Mountains 荆山 and the Yellow River, near the Luo River 洛水 area. This fits with arguments regarding the actual location of a possible Chuan River.[39] Furthermore, associating themselves with the mythology of a powerful Shang king, the Chu may have been co-opting access to a local god, associated with city of Shangqiu 商丘 in the former state of Song, presumably populated by Shang descendants. By the time the *Chu ju* was written, Song had already been absorbed by Chu. Earlier, during the Spring and Autumn period, Pan Geng was worshipped in the state of Song at the west gate for protection against fire.[40] Originally, the Song region was simply a buffer between the strong states of Chu and Qi. As the Chu government was pressed into this region by the advancing Qin army, perhaps an ancestral link to a local deity became imperative when negotiating with the powerful families of the state of Qi. An earlier minister in Qi, named Shu Yi 叔夷, claimed a lineage relationship back to the Shang (for this reason, later scholars assume he must have come from the Song 宋, the state according to legend reserved by the Zhou for the Shang descendants to worship their ancestors). The Shu Yi bell inscriptions dated to the late Spring and Autumn period and trace his lineage back to the first founder Cheng Tang 成湯, presumably many generations earlier than Pan Geng.[41]

Unfortunately, we do not know where the Tsinghua bamboo books come from and hence cannot correlate the location of their burial with the movement of the Chu state. The writing style of the books and the fact that they were preserved at all suggests that they, like the Guodian and Shanghai Museum bamboo texts, derived from a tomb near the Warring States Chu metropolis Jiangling in the upper middle Yangzi River valley, or, at least, somewhere in modern Hubei. A more western location of the text weakens the argument that the text was written purely for political propaganda purposes, as we have no idea what connection a person in Jiangling would have with the push east. On the other hand, these texts were probably written not long before the Qin army overran the Chu capital in 278 BCE.

Nevertheless, we cannot prove that the Chu always believed their history traced back to the Shang. Earlier scholars, such as Rao Zongyi 饒宗頤, relying on transmitted texts suggested that the "split side" births in Chu genealogical accounts must be western, not eastern. Huangfu Mi connected the divine birth to the astral house of Mao 昴, linked more often with the northwest and winter. Rao suggested that the myths of gods born of split-side births might be traced back to South Asian

Indian culture, where similar myths can found in the Rigveda, a text presumably written in India around the same time that oracle bones were being used at Yinxu. Indra in this text grew to a great size immediately upon birth from his mother's side. The tale of the birth of Buddha was similar to *Zigao* tales of Yu and Xie's abilities to talk immediately after birth, except that Buddha was able to walk. Coincidently, in the tale of the birth of Buddha (possibly known as early as the Han dynasty), like the sacrifice at the Pian-wood hut mentioned in the *Chu ju*, discussed earlier, such a birth could only take place at night.[42]

Rao speculated that the Gui people who provided the wife for Lu Zhong were actually Xia peoples and that Yu of the Xia period arose among the Western Qiang peoples. Hence, he concluded that such tales must have flowed into the central Xia region from the Qiang Rong peoples.[43] However, present evidence now suggests an eastern bias, although the geographical origins of Chu people and the history of the "split-side" birthing tale may never be known. At minimum, we do know that difficult births requiring outside intervention were not unknown in the ancient world, so it is entirely possible that the Chinese versions are completely indigenous. The survival of the baby may have seemed a product of divine aid. Surely, when the Zhou myth of the birth of Hou Ji was recorded, the "split-side" birth style was already a possibility and by the late Warring States period was well known in myth if not in daily experience.

Conclusion

In ancient China, as in many traditional cultures that were struggling to survive and expand, birthing was a critical topic. Although men in hierarchal societies generally occupied the most powerful political positions, they still relied on women to give them heirs. Thus, state diviners and shaman-doctors monitored the birthing by royal women. The mystery of life emerging from the body of women became a metaphor for the birth of the cosmos as well. Their connection to the divine, as portal between life and eternity, gave the mothers of a people or of state founder deities a special status. As with the divine kings who received their orders from Heaven, referred to as the Sons of Heaven 天子, these women, likewise, were not impregnated by ordinary men. They did so by visiting magical sites, picking phallic herbs, and mixing with gods.

The *Chu ju* represents a version of this tale with the added twist of the "split-side birth." As we know, an especially strong male agent mixing with a strong female agent can produce traumatic results, but, in the cases of the founders of non-Zhou states, such trauma ironically indicates an auspicious birth. The mother may return to Heaven, but the child will go on to rule. In the case of the Chu state, which rose to prominence after the fall of the Zhou, the goal to create an empire was to fail until a man of the fallen Chu region finally arose and created the Han dynasty in 206 BCE. It is no wonder that we hear that it was a dragon at the edge of a Great Swamp who impregnated this man's mother.[1]

Notes

Introduction

1. The importance of women in social reproduction is clearly recognized in Qin and Han law. See Cui Mailing and Zhang Rongfang 2005, 10–11.

2. Compare the medical texts available for analysis in Bray 1997, 273–368; Furth 1999; Yates 2005; Leung 2006; Wu 2010.

3. Li Xueqin 2010–2016, vol. 1, 115–124, vol. 2, 180–194. For details, see discussion and notes in chapter 5.

Chapter 1. Words and Images

1. Oracle bone forms are adapted from Yu Xingwu 1996 and Yao Xiaosui and Xiao Ding 1989. Bronze images come from Institute of History and Philology, Academia Sinica. For the Shang word *ren*, see discussion by Keightley 2012, 50–51, 58.

2. Yao Xiaosui and Xiao Ding 1989, vol. 1, 15; Keightley 1999, 33. See also notes on this in Peng Bangjiong 2006, 6. Pregnancy in the "Da Ming" 大明 ode in the *Shijing* was referred to as *you shen* 有身.

3. Zhongguo shehui kexueyuan kaogu yanjiusuo 1984–1994, vol. 63; hereafter, *Jicheng* plus the number of the inscription (e.g., *Jicheng* 63).

4. Phonetic reconstructions follow Baxter-Sagart Old Chinese reconstruction in Baxter and Sagart 2014. For a description of the idea of the body beginning in the fourth century BCE, see Lewis 2006a, 13–76. For the body as a pregnant body, see Pu Maozuo 2001.

5. Liang Qing and Xie Xiuying 2001; Pu Maozuo 2001; Zhao Pingan 2001; Qiu Xigui 1993, 1998. For prayers to the Chu founder ancestor named Yu 粥 or 鬻, a frequent loan word with *yu* "to produce, birth" (both pronounced *m-quk), see C. A. Cook 2006, 100. The graph representing this semi-mythical founder of the Chu people was anciently associated with cooked sacrificial offerings.

The fact that it can also be read as "birth" or "birth-ancestor" is suggestive, but we have no proof of this word as a name of an ancestor until Warring States time, see chapter 6 discussion. Takashima 2010, vol. 2, 587–589. He reads Wu Yu 五毓 as Wu Hou 五后 "the Five Sovereigns," *yu* as "to breed," and *mian* as "parturition." Liu Huan (2010) suggests that *yu* in the oracle bones was in fact a loan for *zhou* 胄 (*lru-s) in the rare sense of "successive generations of junior lineage members." He also notes the possible use of *yu* in the early Zhou bronze inscription, the Ban *gui* 班簋, before the appearance of King Wen's name to indicate his lineage relationship to Mao Ban. Liu produces many intriguing examples, but unfortunately the two words do not seem to have been closely pronounced in later times. We do not know what the Shang-period pronunciations may have been. Huang Guohui explains that in the Shang kinship system the *yu* indicated the "offspring, lower generations" versus those "high ancestors," the *gaozu* 高祖 (2012, 11–15).

6. See Chen Wei 2008.

7. According to "Sigan" 斯干, an ode in the "Xiao Ya" section of the *Shijing*, dreams about bears were omens of the birth of sons, and snakes the omens of girls, see *Shijing zhengyi* 38.309 (*Shisanjing zhushu* edition). For a study of Chu inscriptions from Anhui where the title "drinker" was first noticed, see C. A. Cook 1990, 523–547. For the definition of a Nai as a three-legged tortoise or dragon, see Lewis 2006b, 103.

8. Henansheng wenwu kaogu yanjiusuo 2003, strips Jia-san 35, 83, 188, 197; Yi-liu 22; Ling 254, 162, 560, 522, 554.

9. See *Jicheng* 2755, 3694, 4438–4439, 577, 6418, 10218.

10. For the Qin inscription, see *Jicheng* 4315. For the Chu word, see Henansheng wenwu kaogu yanjiusuo 2003 190, strip 35,

11. Li Xueqin 1988. For the female persona of Yu Yin and an early examination of the 虫 phonetic in both the "Yu" of Yu Yin and "Rong" of Zhu Rong, see C. A. Cook 1994. Hu Houxuan, in his seminal essay claiming that the Chu came from the East, used the argument that Zhu Rong (*tuk luŋ, equivalent to Lu Zhong 陸終 *ruk tuŋ) and the Li 黎 (*rˤij) were associated with the East (1934, 27); see also Su Jianzhou 2009.

12. Li Jiahao 2010.

13. *Liji zhengyi*, "Yueji 樂記," 38.1537 (*Shisanjing zhushu*). In the Fangmatan *Rishu*, the gender of animals and humans are both factors to consider in divination over their welfare. See Gansusheng wenwu kaogu yanjiusuo 2009, 89, 297. For the gendered nature of music, see pp. 334, 297.

14. By the Han period, the vagina was called the "square canister" (*kuang* 筐). Earlier, it was the "fish basket" (*gou* 笱), fish being symbolic of the male. See discussion by Harper 1987, 570–572.

15. Yao Xiaosui and Xiao Ding 1989, vol. 2, 581–582, 782–786. The word "source" (*yuan* 原, *ŋʷar) and "spring" (*quan* 泉, *s-N-ɢʷar) are closer to each other than to "special sacrificial animal" (*lao* 牢, *r.ŋˤaw).

16. Jia Wen (2001) suggests "curved" *wan* 宛 *ʔorʔ, which could be a Han-period loan word for a storage receptacle.

17. See review of arguments on the word *ming* by Jia Wen (2001). Jia suggests that women may have given birth outside at first. Zhao Pingan (2001; 2009, 47–55) also reviews the scholarship. In his 2009 discussion, he links the ancient Shang graph to two variant graphs found in Chu bamboo texts with 元 or 丿 elements written on top of 子 and claims they come from a completely different paleographic lineage than 娩.

18. Harper 1998, 378; Ma Jixing 1992, 780–781.

19. Yao Xiaosui and Xiao Ding 1989, vol. 1, 500–502; Allan 1997, 96–101. The word *sheng* also appears in divination statements indicating which ancestral spirits (out of a pantheon) one began with to present prayers and sacrifices.

20. It is possible that other evidence has been overlooked. Pregnant female torsos in clay were found in an early Neolithic site in Fufeng, Shaanxi. See Xibei daxue wenbo xueyuan kaogu zhuanye 2000, 109–111. Guolong Lai has recently noted the discovery at Houtaizi in Luanping County, Hebei, of seven stone sculptures depicting women giving birth in squatting positions dated to the Neolithic era (2015, 100, fig. 3.1).

21. Neolithic clay phalluses are called *taozu* 陶祖 by archaeologists and found in Yangshao sites in Gansu, Shaanxi, and in sites belonging to Miaodigou 2 culture in Shaanxi, and Yangshao sites in Henan.

22. Dematté 1994; Cook and Major 1999, 132–133; Li Jia 2012. See also symbols of life and death in Li Binghai 2007 and fertility worship in the *Shijing* in Li Hong 2001.

23. Dexter and Mair 2010. Another possible interpretation of this stone sculpture is that she is squatting to give birth rather than displaying her genitals.

24. Wang Yunzhi (2001) suggests that the archaic graph 毓 *m-quk evolved to represent a special graph for a ruler. Later a variant of the graph evolved into 育. The archaic graph for 后 *ɢˤoʔ depicted with a 口 and 婦 represented a royal consort. By the late Zhou period, Hou took over to represent the name of a ruler and at the same time was used for 司 *s-lə. Yin Shengping notes that the title *si* 司 (related to the term *si* 嗣) was added to "mothers'" names on inscribed bronze dedications to reveal their role in the production of the lineage heir (2012, 321–328). The second hexagram in the Shanghai Museum version of the *Zhouyi* is called *si* and written with a 司 over a 子, suggesting an heir. It was equivalent to the Xu 需 hexagram (explained as clouds in the sky, Yin overtaking Yang) in the transmitted version. In the Mawangdui silk manuscript versions, it was written as 需 with either a "clothing" 衣 or "female" 女 semantic element (Ding Sixin 2011, 7).

25. Allan 1991. The term *ya* was also a common title for an official in the Shang government and, by the Western Zhou period, clearly referred to heads of lineages secondary to a central lineage (descended directly from the founder).

26. See Childs-Johnson 1998, 2002, 2008; Wang Qiang 2014; Allan 1991, fig. 36, 40–45; 2010; Ai Lan 2010.

27. Yates 2005, 150–151, 157n98.

28. For the *ding* handle, see the Simu Wu *ding* 司母戊鼎. See also the fetal body emerging from the mouth of the double-bodied tiger on covering two sides of the alcoholic brew container called the Hu *zun* 虎尊 and discovered in 1957 in Funan 阜南 district of Anhui. Compare with the famous alcohol-serving vessel, the Hu shi ren *you* 虎食人卣 from Changsha (see fig. 7). For explanations of this type of imagery for use in shamanistic rituals of transcendence, see Childs-Johnson 2002, 15–24; Allan 1991, 2010; Ai Lan 2010, 174, 184, 192–195. See also Jiang Linchang and Sun Jin 2012, 301, especially the painted pottery from Neolithic Majiayao 馬家窰 culture in Gansu (fig. 3). One figure (fig. 3.c) shows a splayed figure with ribs and vagina displayed.

Chapter 2. Controlling Reproduction: Fertility Prayers

1. Guo Moruo et al. 1978–1982, vol. 1, 17. (Also referred to as *Heji*, followed by the rubbing number.)

2. Peng Bangjiong 2006. See Guo Moruo et al. 1978–1982, vol. 5, 1973, 1976.

3. Guo Moruo et al. 1978–1982, rubbing numbers 34080–34083; Hu Houxuan 2002, 113.

4. *Heji* 2400, *Hebu* 4153 (see Peng Bangjiong et al. 1999).

5. Guo Moruo et al. 1978–1982, vol. 5.

6. Peng Bangjiong 2006, 5–6. *Heji* 21071, 21207 (for inscriptions with *you yun*). See the sixteen examples with *you zi* in Peng Bangjiong 2006, 6.

7. The Di found in oracle bones and bronze inscriptions do not seem to concern themselves with birthing. In those materials, this Di is not found in association with the birth of individuals but rather with more global concerns such as the weather, the directions, settlements, or the ritual affairs of the ruling lineage.

8. *Hebu* 6842.

9. *Jicheng* 2768.

10. *Jicheng* 4331.

11. *Jicheng* 5993.

12. *Jicheng* 4459.

13. Xu Zhongshu 1936; Jin Xinzhou 2006; Deng Peiling 2011.

14. See studies by Huang Guangwu 1992; Chen Yingjie 2008, vol. 2, 654–683.

15. See Deng Peiling 2011, 208.

16. Shandong daxue lishi wenhua xueyuan kaoguxi 1998, 21, 23, fig. 5.

17. This is most likely a description of the vessel rather than of the bride, although there may be purposeful ambiguity. Such binomial reduplicative expressions described the bells or vessels when the ancestral blessings were descending or prayers were going up.

18. *Jicheng* 04645; Guo Moruo 1999, 212

19. *Jicheng* 10280.

20. Wu Zhenfeng 2013.

21. *Jicheng* 6010, 10171. Liu Hehui believes that this woman, Da Meng Ji ("Grand Eldest Ji-lineage woman"), was a woman of Cai referred to in the *Shiji* and *Zuozhuan*. In these accounts, she was first married to King Ping of Chu, but she ran away back to her home in Cai when he became enamored of a young woman from Qin. Her marriage to the Wu king would then have been a second marriage, and Liu suspects that both she and the king were both in their forties. From the *Zuozhuan* (Zhao 19), we see recorded that when King Ping of Chu was still a prince, he was in Cai and took up with a woman from Juyang *feng* who bore him a son who would become his heir when he returned to Chu and became king. The boy had two tutors, the lower-ranked one, Fei Wuji, did not like the heir and so convinced the king to get a wife for him. After the king met with Qin, Wuji then escorted the bride back. But he urged the king to take her himself. So, in the first month of his reign, the Ying-lineage woman from Qin became his wife (楚子之在蔡也, 郹陽封人之女奔之, 生大子建, 及即位, 使伍奢為之師, 費無極為少師, 無寵焉, 欲譖諸王, 曰, 建可室矣, 王為之聘於秦, 無極與逆, 勸王取之, 正月, 楚夫人嬴氏至自秦). We know that she returned to Cai because later in Zhao 23, there is a record that "the mother of the Chu heir Jian was in the Cai town of Ju and she summoned Wu people and instigated for them (to continue fighting against the Chu). This was when the Wu king was still Liao. His heir, Zhufan, entered Ju, took the Chu wife and all her treasures, and returned to Wu. The Chu general, who had already been defeated once, hung himself in shame since he couldn't retrieve her" 楚大子建之母在郹, 召吳人而啟之, 冬, 十月, 甲申, 吳大子諸樊入郹, 取楚夫人, 與其寶器以歸, 楚司馬薳越追之, 不及, 將死, 眾曰, 請遂伐吳以徼之, 薳越曰, 再敗君師, 死且有罪, 亡君夫人, 不可以莫之死也, 乃縊於薳澨.

Liu believes that her dowry vessels ended up in the Cai lord's tomb for several possible reasons. One was the reason suggested by others just discussed and another is the political disruption caused by wars between Wu and Chu that put Cai in an awkward political position (bells inscribed with a loyalty oath to Chu were also found in his tomb). So, Liu speculates that either the vessels never left Cai or Da Meng Ji came home again with her vessels and buried them in Zhao Hou's tomb as a memorial. See Ma Chengyuan et al. 1986–1988, inscription no. 589; Cao Zhaolan 2004, 220–224; Chen Mengjia 1963; Guo Ruoyu 1982; Falkenhausen 1999, 523–525; Falkenhausen 2006, 266–267; Li Xueqin 1989, 160–165; Liu Hehui 1989; *Shouxian Cai Hou mu chutu yiwu* 1956;

Wang Hui 2006, 290–294; Wang Rencong 1985; Yin Difei 1984; Yu Xingwu 1979; Zhu Zhenlei 2005–2006.

22. Some speculate that the reason the daughter's vessels were placed in the Cai Lord's tomb had to do with this murder. Even so, the marriage was odd because both Cai and Wu were both Ji-lineage states. Their marriage would theoretically break a taboo against marriages between the members bearing the same lineage name. Some scholars claim that in fact Cai Zhao Hou and Wu king Guang simply exchanged daughters as part of their alliance to defeat Chu. They think the *Shiji* dating for the first year of the Cai Lord should be 515 BCE, the same year that Wu king Guang came to power. Zhu Zhenlei reviews the debate over dating in his dissertation (2005–2006, 24–25).

23. The original graph has a 示 semantic. In the inscriptions, most occurrences of *zhi* 陟 are followed by *jiang* 降. The combination is quite common in the *Shijing* and elsewhere in the transmitted texts. However, the ancient graph is closest to a variant of *fou* 否 (*pəʔ), which cannot be a loan for *jiang* (*kˤruŋ-s). Scholars recommend the closer loan *fu* "to spread" 敷 (*pʰra), as in "to spread the mandate to the Four Regions." Support for this loan is found in the Middle Western Zhou Shi Qiang *pan* (*Jicheng* 10175): "Shangdi sends down fine *de* as a great protection, spreading all over above and below" 上帝降懿德大屏, 匍有上下. The late Western Zhou-period Mao Gong *ding* 毛公鼎 (*Jicheng* 2841) has a different usage: "[I, the king,] command you to manage the domestic and outside affairs of our state and home. Rely on the smaller and larger government structures to protect my throne, so (those) frightening and tricky (spirits) above and below (send) blessings spreading all over the Four Regions, so nothing disturbs the throne of me, The Lone One. Guide me with your knowledge" 命汝乂我邦、我家內外, 憃 (擁) 于小大政, 屏朕位, 虩 (赫) 許 (戲) 上下若否 (敷) 于四方, 死 (尸) 毋 (毋) 童 (動) 余一人在位, 引唯乃智 (知). The early Chunqiu Zhejiang *zhong* 者減鐘 (*Jicheng* 197) has an expression similar to the Cai vessel but describes the rise and fall of a bell sound: "it ascends to (those) sprits above and below and is heard throughout the Four Regions" 其登于上下, 聞于四旁 (方).

24. In late Western Zhou and Chunqiu bronze inscriptions, the graph 害 is sometimes used for words usually written as *gai* 匄, *he* 曷, or *wu* 吾. All were near homophones.

25. See Chen Jian 2001. Cai Wei (2009) suggests there are some variants of the archaic graph *shen* 慎 that could be read as a loan for *shen* 神.

26. Note the wedding song "Wei yang" 渭陽 in the Qin section of the *Shijing* with the phrase 悠悠我思 "far away are my thoughts"; it seems to be a boy who is being escorted in this song (Kong Yingda 1980, herein referred to as *Maoshi zhengyi* 6.106). Some scholars suggest 優優 described the harmonious spread of good government; others that 優遊 described leisurely or soft and harmonious movement. Both terms are found in the *Shijing*.

27. *Jicheng* 00277, 00278.

28. Tian was a space (the sky) with supernatural agency. Shangdi may have originally represented one or multiple High Gods, possibly distant ancestral

deities perceived as having ascended into the sky (see discussion by Allan 2007). Chen Mengjia (1988, 580–581), on the other hand, felt there is no connection between Di and Shang royal ancestors. Di was a term applied to dead kings by the Shang as a religious designation for worship in the ancestral shrines. During the late Zhou era, it was also applied to prehistorical sage-kings. The Qin emperor adopted it along with the typical ancestral epithet "Brilliant, August" (*huang* 皇) as a living title, *huangdi*, for the emperor.

29. See discussion in Ke Heli 2016.
30. See C. A. Cook 2009.
31. *Maoshi zhengyi* 17.528.
32. See Allan 2009, 135–136.
33. Wang Yinzhi 2000, 86. Some scholars suggest that instead of reading the graph *dong* 冬 as *zhong* 終, a common graphic loan in inscriptions and in bamboo texts, that it should be understood as "winter" (*dong*). However, from our examination of the Gaomei fertility rite and of the correlation of spring with birthing, this explanation is unlikely. Both Ma Chengyuan (2001–2011, vol. 2 197) and Wang Yinzhi understand it to mean "already, finally."
34. The graph *li* 吏 is read as *shi* 使 elsewhere in the *Zigao* (see strip 8). The missing graphs are filled in according to other records of the legend and a partial 子 graph is evident. The word *shang* 尚 in the prayer *shang shi zi* 尚吏 (使) 子 is understood as "perhaps" or "making something more approximate" (庶几也, see the *Erya zhushu* 3.15).
35. See Ma Chengyuan's commentary on *Zigao* strips 12–13 (2001–2011, vol. 2, 197–198). Note that strip 12 is incomplete so that there is a break in the narrative before strip 13.
36. Takikawa 1977, 4.2.
37. Wen Yiduo 2005 (originally published in 1935); Chen Mengjia 1937.
38. Zhang Fuhai (2003) suggests that "Chuanjiu" should be read as "Dark Building" (Xuangong 玄宮). Bai Yulan (2003) prefers "Dark Hill" (Xuangqiu 玄丘).
39. Wen Yiduo 2005, 860–863.
40. Granet 1919, 164–165.
41. The song "Summoning the Soul" 招魂 notes: "Cloud-soul! Come back! Do not descend to that Gloomy Capital" 魂兮歸來, 君無下此幽都些. Wang Yi 王逸 (ca. CE 89–158) explains that "the Gloomy Capital, is under the earth and governed by Houtu (the earth god). Under the earth it is gloomy and dark, so it is named the Gloomy Capital" 幽都, 地下后土所治也. 地下幽冥, 故稱幽都 (*Cuci buzhu* 9.5). In later Daoist ritual, this "dark" color was also associated with the internal "mother" spirit employed by the male acolytes to birth their inner embryo (Raz 2014, 191).
42. *Liji zhengyi, Shisanjing zhushu*, 1361.
43. In the *Shijing* ode "Changfa" 長發: "There was Song who was favored and Di who set up her son to create the Shang" 有娀方將、帝立子生商 (*Maoshi zhengyi* 20. 626). See also "Dark Bird" (*Maoshi zheng yi* 20. 622–623).

44. See "Tian Wen" 天問 (*Chuci buzhu* 3.16); "Yin benji" 殷本紀 (Takikawa, 3.2); see also comments in Sukhu 2012, 52–53, 222–230n53.

45. Granet 1919, 470–471.

46. "Liyi zhi" 禮儀志, *Hou Han shu*, 3107. Quoting from the "Yueling zhangju" 月令章句.

47. "Liyi zhi" 禮儀志, *Hou Han shu*, 3108.

48. The words gao 梟 (*kˤu) and gao 高 (*Cə.kˤaw) were used as loans for each other. Wang Yinzhi (2000, 336) claimed that the Gaomei 高禖 in the "Yueling" was Jiaomei 郊禖, claiming that gao was a loan for jiao (*kˤaw).

49. *Maoshi zhengyi* 17.528.

50. Granet interprets this as a purification ritual used by childless women to get rid of bad luck (1919, 165).

51. *Maoshi zhengyi* 17.528.

52. See the Bin Gong xu, C. A. Cook 2012–2013. Granet notes that *de* shared by members of the same clan was one reason behind the social rule that people of the same clan name should not marry (1919, 208–209).

53. *Maoshi zhengyi* 20.614.

54. *Zhouli zhushu* 22.789.

55. Ma Ruichen 1989, 1139.

56. Chen Shouqi 1988, 7,150. For the *Shuowen* definition, see Duan Yucai 1988, 7.

57. Chen Huan 1988, 1170

58. Sun Zuoyun 1966, 298. Sun felt that the Bigong and Mei divinity derived from an ancestress god into a marriage and fertility goddess.

59. Granet 1919, 157–165, 470–471, 178, 217–220; 1926, 321, 428–441, 457–465.

60. *Zhouli zhushu* 14, 733.

61. Li Fengxiang 2004, 1034.

62. Chen Qiyou 2002, 68.

63. Wu Yujiang 2006, 338.

64. See Guo Moruo 1982, 9 ("Shi zu bi" 釋祖妣, Guo Moruo quanji, "Kaogu bian" 考古編, juan 1); Wen Yiduo 2005, 83–85.

65. *Chunqiu zuozhuan zhengyi* 3.1723.

66. Duan Yucai 1988, 194.

67. Wen Yiduo 2005, 108; Sun Zuoyun 1966, 300–301.

68. *Maoshi zhengyi* 17.528.

69. *Maoshi zhengyi* 17.528.

70. Xu Lianggao, 1999, 254. See also n. 24.

71. "Liyi zhi" 禮儀志, *Sui shu*, 146.

72. He Yaohua 1982.

73. *Maoshi zhengyi* 17.528.

74. "Kongzi shijia" 孔子世家, *Shiji*, 1905.

75. Zhu Xi 2001, 42; Yuan Ke 1985, 212.

76. See Yan Ruxian and Song Zhaolin 1983, 207.

77. Yuan Ke 1985, 2.
78. Yuan Ke 1985, 28.
79. Yuan Ke 1985, 115.
80. From Shuihudi, Liu Lexian 1993, 230.

Chapter 3. Mothers and Embryos

1. For a recent discussion of ritual reform in the second half of the Western Zhou period, see Falkenhausen 2006, chapter 1. For a discussion of "appointment" rituals (of which promotion rituals for heirs constitute a subsection), see F. Li 2008, 105–110; see also C. A. Cook 2017.

2. The connection between these two gods was made by David Pankenier (2004) and Sarah Allan (2007) in separate studies.

3. Some suggest that *di* was a loan for the homophone *di* 嫡 "son of the principal wife" (see Qiu Xigui 2012, 124).

4. See discussions in Allan 1997, 2003; Harper 2001. See also the summary of scholarly debate presented in S. Cook 2012, vol. 1, 323–341.

5. Cao Feng 2011. The Guodian version of the *Laozi* has a similar sentence: 周行無怠; comparative texts can be found in S. Cook 2012, vol. 1; Henricks 2000; Ai Lan and Wei Kebin 2002; Ding Sixin 2010.

6. S. Cook 2012, 347–348. *Taiyi sheng shui* strips 6–7.

7. The feminine nature of the Dao has been a source of much discussion, see K. Lai 2000; Xie 2000; L. Ma 2009, 2012; R. Wang 2003; Liu Xiaogan 2003; Hall and Ames 2000; Goldin 2000; Raphals 1998, 140–141; C. Despeux and L. Kohn 2003, 7–13; Liu Xiaogan 2006, 93–94, 136–141, 317–321, 440–442, 517–518, 585–588, 716–720.

8. See C. A. Cook and Zhao Lu, 2017.

9. *Xunzi jijie* 18.316–317; Knoblock 1994, vol. 3, 199.

10. *Xunzi jijie* 13.251; Knoblock 1994, vol. 3, 73.

11. S. Cook 2012, vol. 1, 348.

12. On the philosophical shape and substance of water, see Allan 1997, 29–61.

13. For a discussion tracing the origins of *yinyang* cosmology to concerns over reproduction and fertility, see Qiao Anshui 2003.

14. S. Cook 2012, vol. 1, 343–346.

15. Li Xueqin 2010–2016, vol. 5, 14–17, 73–83, 141–148 (*Qinghua daxue cang Zhan guo zhujian*); for Yi Yin, see Allan 2015 ("'When Red Pigeons Gather'").

16. For a complete study of this practice and its Western Zhou origins, see C. A. Cook 2017 (*Ancestors, Kings, and the Dao*).

17. Raz 2014.

18. The standard translation of this name as "queen mother" is a misnomer. In pre-Qin excavated texts a *wangmu* was a female ancestor older than one's father.

19. Raz 2014, 131.
20. Divine tortoises were used in Han divination.
21. Raz 2014, 192.
22. Raz 2014, 192.
23. See Li Xueqin 2010–2016, vol. 5, 148.
24. By twelve weeks into a pregnancy, the fetus fills the uterus.
25. Bones develop around the thirteenth week.
26. Gender identification is actually possible at fourteen weeks.
27. There is still much debate over the individual readings of the archaic graphs. We have simply presented one likely reading based on the rhyme pattern and the most likely loan words.
28. Raz 2014, 186–187 (table 7.1).
29. Harper 1998, 372–385.
30. The relevant section of text from the chapter "Jingshen xun" 精神訓 is found in Li Xueqin 2010–2016, vol. 5, 148.
31. The relevant section of text from the chapter "Jiu shou" 九守 is found in Li Xueqin 2010–2016, vol. 5, 148.
32. Muscles appear in week 13.
33. Tendons grow in the seventh week.
34. Movement of a fetus can be felt variously between the sixteenth and twentieth weeks of pregnancy.
35. At the fourteenth week the entire body of the fetus begins to be covered by a fine hair; only by the thirtieth week does longer hair begin to grow on its head.
36. The eyes open around the twenty-sixth week.

Chapter 4. Controlling the Pregnant Body

1. A mystery word often found in hunting divination and interpreted by some as a verb meaning to "pursue" an animal. The meaning here is uncertain. Perhaps it is a mistake for a Bing 丙 day.
2. Keightley 1999.
3. *Heji* 6948 front, 14128 back.
4. Yao Xiaosui and Xiao Ding 1989, 15, 73, 782–785. For a brief review of some of these records, see Li Min 1993, 246–249. For shamans working with fertility and childbirth issues, see Zhao Rongjun 2011, 95–101.
5. Liu Lexian 1993, 69–72; 2012, 49–50. For a complete description of the many varied and complex calendar systems recorded for the Warring States, Qin, and Han periods, but particularly as reflected in the *Day Books*, see Harper and Kalinowski, forthcoming, chapter 4.
6. Tianshui Fangmatan in Gansusheng wenwu kaogu yanjiusuo 2009, 1–2, 89, 91, 123, 125. For the association with the sun, 16, 412–413.
7. Liu Lexian 1993, 69–72, 291–292.

8. Ibid., 165–168; Dai Nianzu 2001.
9. Liu Lexian 1993, 21–31. See also Harper and Kalinowski, forthcoming.
10. Liu Lexian 1993, 31–41, 53–60.
11. Liu Lexian 2012, 50, strips 16–17, 19.
12. Li Xueqin 2010–2016, vol. 4. For a full discussion and translation of the *Shifa*, see C. A. Cook and Zhao Lu, 2017.
13. In the *Shifa* any set of trigrams that are opposite each other in line type, such as Qian and Kun, are considered husband-and-wife pairs.
14. See C. A. Cook and Zhao Lu, 2017.
15. Lin Zhongjun 2014.
16. Diviners analyzed the trigrams in the *Shifa* in sets of four, two on top and two on bottom. See C. A. Cook and Zhao Lu 2017. Note that "wash water" was a metaphor for licentious male behavior that results in *gu* 蠱 poisoning. See Ke Heli 2016.
17. Shuihudi Qin mu zhujian zhengli xiaozu 1990, 206. Similar diagrams are found later in materials such as those found in the Mawangdui *Taichan shu*. See Ma Jixing 1993, 779–814; Harper 1998, 372–384. For discussion and comparison to later manuals, see Hinrichs and Barnes 2013, 70–75.
18. Shuihudi *Rishu* Yi 乙, strip 247.
19. Shuihudi *Rishu* Jia 甲, strip 145.
20. The movement of the spirit to different sites inside the body is suggested by Rao Zongyi based on later texts and contested by Liu Lexian (1993, 187–191).
21. For a discussion of marriage and sexuality related lines in the *Zhouyi*, see Shaughnessy 1992, 1995. Infertility for specific time periods, such as three or ten years, are mentioned in hexagrams Chun 純 and Jian 漸.
22. C. A. Cook 2006, 91–97; Yan Changgui 2010.
23. It is unlikely that the Baoshan text was referring to the Tai Yin channel of the body mentioned in early imperial-era medical texts.
24. These two may have been gendered (see the discussion in Ke Heli 2016). In the Shuihudi *Day Book*, fields were supervised by the supernatural hierarchy of Field Ancestor (*tianzu* 田祖), Field Father (*tianfu* 田父), and Field Mother (*tianmu* 田母) (see Liu Lexian 1993, 47–48).
25. See the case of Shao Tuo examined in Ke Heli 2016.
26. Li Xueqin 2010–2016, vol. 4, 115.
27. A description of people occupying the Center (versus other cosmic directions) listed in the "Zhuixing xun" 墜形訓 chapter of the *Huainanzi* (146) lists someone with a large face and small neck along with other deformities.
28. Li Xueqin 2010–2016, vol. 4, 117n21. In the almanacs, becoming a shaman (male *xi* 覡 or female *wu* 巫) is the fate of children born on certain days.
29. Ibid., 109–116, 193.
30. Li Xueqin 2010–2016, vol. 4, 109–116, 193. Childs-Johnson 2008 discusses the relationship between shamans and the practice of *yi*, a kind of spiritual metamorphoses represented in Shang animal mask iconography.

31. Shuihudi Qin mu zhujian zhengli xiaozu 2001, 181–192, 214, 231, 234, 237–238; see especially the "Sheng zi" 生子 chapter, 202–205, 251–254; Liu Lexian 1993, 229–230; Liu Tseng-kuei 2009, 908–914.

32. Harper 1998, 379.

33. This may have been a type of insect. Ma Jixing 1993, 806; Harper 1998, 381n7.

34. On *hun* and *po*, see Poo 1998, 62–66, 163–165; Brashier 2011, 253–254, 417n67. For a discussion of the sequestering of birthing women because of bodily fluids, see Kinney 2004, 167–168; Song Jie 2009. For leaking during pregnancy, see Yinqueshan Hanmu zhujian zhengli xiaozu 2010, vol. 2, 225.

35. Zhao 29 in *Chunqiu Zuozhuan zhengyi* 53.420.

36. *Liji zhengyi* 28.1469 ("Neize" 內則). For a review of transmitted textual records on birthing, see Qi Wenxin 1998, 402–403.

37. Yao Xiaosui and Xiao Ding 1989, 742–743, see *Heji* 14017; 509, 742–743; see *Heji* 8043, 8044 正, 14017 正, 1550, 722 正, 8041, 33134, 33135.

38. There are many attempts to date Ji Lian and the other figures mentioned in the text. See, for example, Yin Hongbing 2013.

39. Fudan University Excavated Text and Paleographical Research Center Graduate Reading Group 2011; Da Haobo (2011) places Jingzong at the head of the Jing Mountains 荊山 in Hubei. See also discussion by Zhou Yunzhong 2013, 229–230, who like others puts Jingzong in the Dan River region of the Qin range.

40. Gao Chongwen 2011, 61–62, 66.

41. Ibid., 62–65. Gao notes that around the time of Zhou king Zhao, who attacked Chu, the Chu leaders were based farther south, across the Han River. He places Ruo, occupied by Xiong Yi, at a place once called Shangmi 商密 in the Dan River valley. He notes that by the end of the Western Zhou period, the Chu people had already populated the Jiang-Han (Yangzi-Han Rivers) region and begun to create their own distinct culture. See also the discussion by Xia Mailing 2013.

42. Lai Guolong connects it to the Han name for a shrine, the *pian fang* 梗房, built within or as part of a tomb (2015, 89–90).

43. Chen Wei 2011.

44. Li Xueqin (2011, 57) suggests that *pian* should be "to roast" *fan* 燔, meaning that the room was built for roasting the calf. He also suggests that "corpse" 尸 should be read as 陳, indicating that the calf was displayed after it was put into the hut. He notes the original Chu graph transcribed "to sacrifice" 祭 was written with a variant of 亦 (for 夜) over 示, a graph used in many Chu month names (see discussion in C. A. Cook 2006, 92–94, esp. table 1 on p. 93).

45. Cook and Major 1999, 56. For a recent exploration of the Ruo people during the Shang period and later, see Shen Jianhua 2012.

46. Seligman et al. 2008, 62–66.

47. Lewis 1990, 44–45, 199.

48. This association may have been a function of sound magic as the ancient words for punishment and *jing* "thorn, briar" were near homophones. See Yinqueshan Hanmu zhujian zhengli xiaozu 2010, vol. 2, 205. For *xing* and *de*, see Major 1987; Kalinowski 1998–1999.

49. Harper notes cognate words that connote "the subjugation of demonic forces by means of exorcistic weapons" (1987, 478). The thorn may have been used in "spellbinding" (*jie* 詰). Peach-wood bows and jujube arrows were shot at demons that inhabited old tombs (Harper 1987, 493).

50. See "Jiaosi zhi" 郊祀志 in the *Hanshu*, 1231; see also Liu Lexian 1993, 257–260.

51. For theories of the role of the thorn, see Liu Xinfang 2013, 124–125. For breach births, see Hinrichs and Barnes 2013, 74; for imperial-era medical records on a variety of methods for difficult births, see Du Lanfang 2012.

52. The original fourteen strips did not have a title, but Li Xueqin noting its similarity to the "Ju pian" 居篇 of the *Shiben* titled it the *Chu ju*, which likewise chronicles the movements of leaders (Li Xueqin 2010–2016, vol. 1, 180). Zhao Pingan (2011) dates the *Chu ju* to Chu king Su's 肅 reign (370–341 BCE). The *Chu ju* narrative of royal residences and major moves ends with King Dao's 悼 reign (384–381 BCE). Other bamboo texts from the same period show the beginnings of the same "X begat Y" rhetorical model with the occasional female added. We see this, for example, in the Tsinghua *Xinian* 繫年, from the same collection as the *Chu ju* and also written in the third century BCE, but the only women mentioned are those, such as Bao Si 褒姒, who birthed kings and caused battles or other diplomatic snafus. The *Xinian* is vol. 2 of the *Qinghua daxue cang Zhanguo zhujian*. See sections 2, 6, and 15 for examples.

Chapter 5. Divine Origins and Chu Genealogical History

1. Harper 1999, 813–884. See Lei Xueqi 1957, 1–6. The *Shiben* begins with the "Three Brilliancies" (San Huang 三皇) sky and earth gods, Tai Hao Fuxi shi and Yandi Shennong shi, before listing Huangdi. The *Shiji* begins with Huangdi. See Takikawa 1977, 40.2–6.

2. Liu Tao (2011) notes other texts where spirits are brought down onto mountains. For a thorough discussion of this religious framework, shamanism, and the *Chuci*, see Sukhu 2012.

3. Luo Xiaohua (2010) shows the connection between the Shang oracle bone graphs (including one with a female semantic element) for "visit" (*bin* 賓) and its descendant graphs in Chu bamboo texts. The meaning of the word varies. It is understood by some as indicative of a spirit or shamanistic journey and others as simply "to join (as mate)" or "to entertain" (see *Heji* 5874). Jiang Linchang and Sun Jin (2012) note that the shamanistic journey symbolically involved sacrificing a young woman to Shangdi. In Ancestress Lie's case, they

claim that since the shaman doctor fixed her up, she must have come back to life. They note a number of similar stories where figures come back to life or are transformed, such as Gun into a yellow bear.

4. For Fu Hao, see the tomb report translated by Childs-Johnson 1983. For Wang Jiang, Jin Jiang, and the Dong *ding*, see *Jicheng* 2704, 4060, 4132–4133, 4300–4301, 5407 (Wang Jiang), 2826 (Jin Jiang), 2789 (Dong).

5. The Shu Yi 叔夷 bells, *Jicheng* 272, 85; for Chen and Ju inscriptions, see *Jicheng* 271, 277, 284, 4145, 4152, 5629, 2630, 4646, 4647. The power of Jiang 姜 women is of special interest to a study of female sociopolitical power but beyond the confines of this essay.

6. Lewis 2006b, 109–116.

7. Cahill 1993.

8. Many scholars have compared the *Chu ju* list to the transmitted textual versions. See, for example, Niu Pengtao 2013.

9. Chen Hou Yinci *dui*, *Jicheng* 4649; Li Ling 1994; C. A. Cook 2009, 270n108.

10. Note that Xuanxu appears as a place-name in the Chu Silk Manuscript and the Xin Cai divination text (Liu Xinfang 2002–2203, 135; Yang Hua 2007, 364, strips Jia 3, 11, 24)

11. The Thunder Deity 雷神 in the "Hainei dong jing" 海內東經 was a dragon with a human head that lived in the Thunder Swamp 雷澤 and drummed on its abdomen (Yuan Ke 1993, 381). In the "Da Huang dong jing" 大荒東經 in the eastern sea near Liu Bo lived a snake-like creature that glistened like the sun and moon and sounded like thunder (Yuan Ke 1993, 416). This creature's name was Kui 夔, the same name mentioned in the "Shundian" of the *Shangshu* as Shun Di's music master. In the "Da Huang dong jing" account, Huangdi made a drum out of the creature's skin, beating it with the bones of the Thunder Beast 雷獸 to frighten everyone below.

12. "Hainei jing" in the *Shanhaijing*. See Yuan Ke 1985, 297.

13. Fudan University Excavated Text and Paleographical Research Center Graduate Reading Group 2011.

14. Takikawa 1977, 1.14–17.

15. Lei Xueqi 1957, 4.

16. Takikawa 1977, 40.2–46.

17. Li Xueqin 2010–2016, vol. 1, 115–124, vol. 2, 180–194; Fudan University Excavated Text and Paleographical Research Center Graduate Reading Group 2011.

18. In numerous Western Zhou inscriptions, the king's position is the first thing remarked after the date and sometimes only the position and not the date. In bamboo texts from the Chu area, we find this in the Baoshan inscriptions (C. A. Cook 2006, 154) and in the first strip of the Shanghai Museum bamboo text "Wang ju" 王居, in Ma Chengyuan 2001–2011, vol. 8, 206–207.

19. Sukhu 2012, 102–104, 144–163, 191, 194.

20. For a discussion of the importance of particular days of the calendar with a male or female birth, see Kinney 2004, 109–111.

21. Li Shoukui points out that in the "Xi shan jing" of *Shanhaijing*, Chu divinity Lao Tong lived on a jade-topped mountain called Gui shan 騩山 (2012, 34). The sacred mountain is written as 嶡山 in the Baoshan divination and sacrifice texts. Chen Wei 1996, 176; C. A. Cook 2006, 7, 101, 110, 115, 174, 175, 199, 202. See also Zhou Yunzhong 2013, 220–225.

22. In the "Wudi benji," Huangdi's son Zhuanxu had a son named "Cave Cicada" (Qiongchan 窮蟬) (Takikawa 1977, 1.17). In the "Da huang xi jing" 大荒西經 of the *Shanhaijing*, Xi Wangmu is recorded as living in a cave (穴處) (Yuan Ke 1993, 16.466). Xu Shaohua (2012) places Ji Lian's early residences in the Dan River region. See also Zhou Yunzhong 2013, 220–225.

23. In the "Wudi benji" of the *Shiji*, Huangdi was buried at Qiao Mountain 橋山 (Takikawa 1977, 1.17). See also Zhou Yunzhong 2013, 220–225.

24. Gao Chongwen notes that most scholars agree that this is the Jun River 均水 (later known as Xichuan 淅川) (2012, 63). See also Zhou Yunzhong 2013, 225–226.

25. See discussion by Zhao Pingan 2012.

26. Shan Zhouyao (2013) after evaluating various readings for this unusual sentence accepts it as a loan for "Ancestress Wei grasping angelica travels all around the realm" 妣隹秉茲率相歷遊四方. Although "angelica" (*zhi*) appears in the *Chuci*, it is never the object of "to grasp" (*bing*). While divination stalks or a pen might be grasped (*bing*), so too is the common idea of "grasping *de*" (*bing de* 秉德), hence, the Qinghua team's reading of "loving kindness" (*ci* 慈), an approved parental virtue especially by the Han period, seems just as likely. The idea of a wandering female is seen in later versions of "split-birth" tales where the mother of Yu, Gun's wife, collects Job's tears in the mountains as part of the Gaomei ritual. The word *li* 署 *C.raj-s is read as either a loan for "beauty" 麗 *rˤe-s or 歷 *rˤek but the words were not as closely pronounced as suggested. It is much closer to "encounter, depart" 離 *raj. The graph written with a 由 over a 日 is assumed to be a loan with the phonetic 由 *lu, possibly 遊 *ɢu, with the obvious graphic loan *zhou* 胄 *lru-s rejected because of its common use as "helmet," military gear being an unlikely accessory for a young girl. Another possibility suggested was "to go to" *di* 迪 *sˤek or *dˤek. The authors temporarily accept the unusual combination of "departing and arriving" (*lidi*) as a reading with the idea that the princess, like her father, had to wander over hill and dale before finding a place to live.

27. Liu Xinfang reads this as "to ask about the time" (*wenqi* 問期) to make sure the day is auspicious (2013, 123–124).

28. There are a number of radically different interpretations for this line. We base our interpretation on the terms *chang* and *xiang*, defined in the *Daodejing* 55 as "harmony" and "abundant production" 知和曰常, 知常曰明, 益生曰祥. The phrase "to cast aside the normal and be inauspicious" 廢常不祥

occurs in the *Zuozhuan* Xiang 19 when a king considered replacing the heir with a favorite concubine's son (*Chunqiu Zuozhuan zhengyi* 1980, 34.1968). See also the use in the *Rishu* Jia strip 11, Shuihudi Qin mu zhujian zhengli xiaozu 2001, 181. Zhao Pingan (2012) follows the original Qinghua commentary but explores further the idea that the phrase describes where the twins were born not how they were born.

29. The Tsinghua editors note that the graph *lie* 列 (*ret) in the *Rong Cheng Shi* was read as *li* 厲 (*rat) ("whetstone") for 癘 ("pestilence, infliction"). This is a possible loan in the Chu dialect, but since we have no other record of this ancestress, it is not necessary. If her name was really Pestilence, then a connection to the Pestilence Ghost in other texts must be made. In the *Zuozhuan* a Li demon appeared in the dreams as a yellow bear associated also with Gun, the father of Sage-King Yu (C. A. Cook 2013, 18–20). Strips 43–46 in the chapter "Jiejiu" of the Shuihudi *Day Book*, on the other hand, explain that the Pestilence ghost comes in the form of a baby (Liu Lexian 1993, 225–268).

30. Han Liu 韓流 is described in the "Hainei jing" 海內經 of the *Shanhaijing* as having small ears and was the dragon-like father of Zhuanxu (Yuan Ke 1993, 18, 503). See also the discussion by Sarah Allan 1991, 67.

31. The reading of the line is somewhat tentative. Two key words are unclear. The graph was interpreted by the Fudan University Excavated Text and Paleographical Research Center Graduate Reading Group as *xian* (*gˤrəm), the name of the shaman, because it is common in other texts to include the name of the shaman after the title *wu* 巫. Shaman Xian appears as a "descending" spirit in the "Lisao" and is associated with shaman-doctors and spirit-mountains in contemporary myth ("Dahuang xi jing" 大荒西經 in *Shanhaijing* and "Zuo pian" 作篇 in *Shiben*), both themes which fit the *Chu ju*. The problem is that the graph was written in an unusual manner with a phonetic that does not seem to match. Some suggest the graph represented a form of *bing* 并 or *jing* 荊, a word meaning either "together" or "thorns, briars," and represented the Chu people (see Liu Tao 2011 for the latter suggestion). Many explain that the graph following Wu 巫 would typically be a name and therefore suggest the variant form ᵚ of the more commonly known Wu Xian 咸. The second key word was the verb *gai* 賅 (該 *kˤə) understood in the rare sense of "to join together." Words with the phonetic *gˤə 亥 are often loaned for *ke* 刻 (*kʰˤək) "to cut." Despite these two uncertainties, we still know that the shaman used thorns to deal with a difficult birth. See discussions in Fudan University Excavated Text and Paleographical Research Center Graduate Reading Group 2011; Liu Tao 2011; Shan Zhouyao 2011, 87–96; Chen Minzhen 2011. According to the *Day Book* A, strip 28, thorns were used to make arrows used in exorcism. See Shuihudi Qin mu zhujian zhengli xiaozu 2001, 212; Liu Lexian 1993, 225–228, 257. Jiang Linchang and Sun Jin (2012) feel that the thorns were used to repair the mother's ribs so that she came back to life after Li Li broke through her ribs. Alternatively, in Qin legal texts the term *he* 劾 meaning to bring a charge by an

official against a suspect (Lau and Staack 2016, 39) can also refer to a magical means of *ming* 命 used to exorcise ghosts (usually in the form of snakes) from sick people and toxic landscapes (see Liu Lexian 1993, 265, and the "Fangshu liezhuan" 方術列傳 of the *Hou Han shu*).

32. *Da Dai Liji jinzhu jinyi*, Gao Ming 1993, 261–262. The graph is considered a depiction of a 羊 and to be the sound of a lamb bleating. It was also considered close to the graph *mou* 牟, the sound of the cow mooing. See Zhu Junsong 1984, 528.

33. Lei Xueqi 1957, 3.

34. Ying Shao 應劭 comp., *Fengsu tongyi* 風俗通義, juan 1 "Huangba, Liu guo" 皇霸·六國, in Wang Liqi 1981, 28.

35. See Pei Yin in Sima Qian 1959, 1690.

36. Concern over the survival of the mother separately and in relation to the child is expressed in the divination text "Xingde xingshi" 刑德行時 from Yinwan, see Zhang Xiancheng and Zhou Junli 2011, 138–139.

37. For a recent discussion of the idea of Sage-King Yu and his father Gun as fish and dragon images, see Lewis 2006b, 19, 103–104, 121, 192n98.

38. Although it is assumed in this tale that the name Chu comes from the original meaning of the graph "thorns," it comes up as a "surname" (*xing* 姓) in a curious entry in the "Sheng zi" 生子 (birthing) chapter of the Shuihudi *Day Book* Yi strip 243: "If you give birth on a Wuxu day, (the baby) will belong to the Chu surname" 戊戌生, 姓楚. This suggests that the surname "Thorns" had more to do with the time of the birth rather than the method. On the other hand, the idea that "thorns" represented a birth outside might be suggested by an entry in the equivalent chapter in *Day Book* Jia, where such a birthday represents "a preference for a settlement or house out in the wilds or fields" 好田野邑室; Shuihudi Qin mu zhujian zhengli xiaozu 2001, 253, 254n4.

39. Zhao Pingan 2013 suggests that these were mis-transcriptions of the archaic graph by later scribes for the names of the two twins of Ji Lian given in the *Chu ju*.

40. Li Xueqin 2010, 55.

41. Ibid., 56.

42. See C. A. Cook 2006, 100, strip 246, following Chen Wei 1996, 238. See also the readings by Huang Xiquan 2006. For discussion of identities of Xue Xiong and Yu Xiong in transmitted texts, see Zhang Fuhai 2010.

43. See discussion on Xiong Li by Meng Pengsheng 2012, 303–307.

Chapter 6. The Traumatic Births of Non-Zhou Ancestors

1. The original graph representing the site for the traumatic birth in the *Chu ju*, for "split-side," is read as *la* 臘 (*rˤap), a loan for *xie* 脅 (*qʰ<r>ep) referring to the ribcage. It becomes a birthing word in the context of split-birth

tales. It is possible that these two words were similar at that time in the Chu dialect. The homophone *la* 拉 meaning "to split" (resulting in having twins) is found in the *Shifa*, see Li Xueqin 2013, vol. 4, 115–116.

2. Li Shoukui (2011) discusses the *Chu ju* version in terms of other versions of Chu founder ancestor myths.

3. See Kinney 2004, 46–48. For a simple account of Hou Ji's "descent and birth" (as a spirit, *jiangsheng* 降生), the fertility ritual, and other rituals employing the popular—but now discounted by modern anthropologists and archaeologists—theories of totems and matriarchy in early society, see Si Weizhi 1997, 50–58. For a review of references to childbirth and herbs in the *Shijing*, see Luo Yuankai 1990.

4. Shi Qiang *pan*, *Jicheng* 10175.

5. Given usage in the *Chu ju*, I suspect the graph read *da* is an ancient mis-transcription for one of the many variant graphs with the 羊 phonetic.

6. Wang Wei (2011) suggests that the Chu split-side birth tale could date no earlier than the second half of the Chunqiu period, maybe later.

7. Found in the "Ming gui, xia" 明鬼下 in *Mozi jiangu*, 247; the "Taishi, shang" 泰誓上 in the *Shangshu zhengyi* 11.180; "Benjing xun" 本經訓 and "Daoyingxun" 道應訓 in *Huainanzi*, 256, 402; "Wang Dao" 王道 in *Chunqiu fanlu*, 106.

8. Liu Xinfang 2013, 124–125.

9. *Jicheng* 5412, 5415.1, 10175, 4498 (the Ersi Bi Qi *you* 二祀邲其卣, the Bao *you* 保卣, the Shi Qiang *pan*, and the Guo Shu *fu* lid 虢叔簠蓋).

10. Yu Xingwu 1993, 321–322. I thank Adam Schwartz for bringing this reference to my attention. See also Hinrichs and Barnes 2013, 74.

11. See Yao Xiaosui and Xiao Ding 1989, 15.

12. The names Baoxi and Fuxi were near homophones. It is unfortunate that the silk manuscript is damaged. Could the female's name have been originally a graphic variation on what was later read as the name of the wife of Lu Zhong, and hence could the origins of the Fuxi-Nüwa coupling also be somehow linked to imagined Chu history? Yuan Wenqing (2008) attempts to explore some of these connections to identify a clear Chu mythology, separating the sky gods from the human ancestors, but also cautions that we must wait for more evidence. He Xin claims that the ancient words for "bear" and "dragon" were homophones (2008, 6–7). According to the Baxter-Sagart reconstruction of the graphs there is little relationship between the words for bear and dragon: 龍 *mə-roŋ, 熊 *C.ɢʷəm {C.(ɢ)ʷrəm}, 能 *nˤə.

13. Some of the graphs in this passage are read slightly differently from that found in Li Ling and C. Cook, "Translation of the Chu Silk Manuscript," in C. A. Cook and J. S. Major 1999, 174. Cf. Li Ling 1985, 64–67; Rao Zongyi and Zeng Xiantong 1985, 4–8. Liu Xinfang adds Nüwa's origins, Sushaqu 夙沙瞿, to the text and reads the line "creating Yu and Xie" 為禹為契 as "creating Snake and Li-demon" 為蛇為厲, claiming that these were nefarious demons that had nothing to do with the four sons of Nüwa (2002–2003, 137–139). See also

He Xin 2008. Cf. analysis of the *Zigao* version by Li Ling 2012. For the *Shiben* reference to Huangdi and the Xiong lineage, see the Lei Xueqi 1957, 2–7.

14. Qiu Xigui 2013.

15. *Shanhaijing jianshu* (Hao Yixing 1974, 479; "Tianwen" 天問 in *Chuci buzhu*, 3.4b–5b; Li Shoukui, Qu bing 曲冰, Sun Weilong 2007, 802. For the definition of a Nai as a three-legged tortoise or dragon, see Lewis 2006b, 103.

16. Ma Chengyuan 2001–2011, vol. 2, 192–197. *Qi*'s birth is recorded on a few bamboo strips preserved at the Chinese University of Hong Kong. See Chen Songzhang 2001, 12; Chen Jian 2003, 56–59, 64; the discussions of the *Zigao* and *Tang Yu zhi dao* by Pines 2005, 254–263; Allan 2009.

17. Allan 2009, 132–136.

18. Found in the "Hainei jing," *Shanhaijing jianshu* (Hao Yixing 1974, 479). For a lengthy discussion of the symbolism of the stone and being born of an evil father, see Lewis 2006b, 102–106, 137–139.

19. Many ritual actions were performed in threes: three hops while mourning, three years of mourning for high-status dead, three performances of the Pace of Yu when entering or exiting gates, three Yin and Yang trigram lines, and so forth. Factors of three are parts of the ritual numbers 6 and 9 found in the *Yijing*.

20. *Shanhaijing jianshu* (Hao Yixing 1974), 479.

21. Yan Kejun 1999, 15, 195; Allan 1991, 70.

22. "Tianwen" in *Chuci buzhu* 1979, 150–152. Trans. Hawkes 1985, 128.

23. See C. A. Cook 2006, 119–147.

24. "Xiuwuxun" 修務訓, in Liu Wendian, 642.

25. See J. Wang 1992. For the stone as associated with fertility, eggs, and Nüwa (Nügua), see 75–78.

26. "Sandai gaizhi, Zhiwen pian" 三代改制, 質文篇, Su Xing 1994, 212; "Qigui pian" 奇怪篇, *Lunheng zhushi*, vol. 1, 217.

27. Gao You commentary on 禹生于石, in Liu Wendian 1989, 642.

28. *Wu Yue Chunqiu* 1996, 44.

29. Huangfu Mi 1998, 21. See Mark Lewis on this passage, 2006b, 19, 103–104.

30. "Wude zhi" 五德志, *Qianfu lun* 8 in Wang Jipei 1985, 393.

31. "Nanman xinan yi liezhuan" 南蠻西南夷列傳, *Hou Han shu* 86, 2829–2930.

32. "Yin benji," Takikawa 1977, 3.16–17. Xie Weiyang (2013) doubts the veracity of any real relationship to Pan Geng.

33. Yang Xiong discussed Yu's birthplace in his *Shuwang benji* 蜀王本紀. See Taiping yulan 82, 1985, vol. 1, 381.

34. Qiu Xigui, 2004, 43.

35. Childs-Johnson 1989, 1998, 2002, 2008; Allan 2010.

36. Fudan University Excavated Text and Paleographical Research Center Graduate Reading Group 5/1/2011 suggests a possible reading of Li 瘋. See also Xu Shaohua 2010, 12–26.

37. See Ross 2000, 433–443, especially 438. In Chu lore, thorns 棘 growing in the Shang court was considered a bad omen for the Shang polity. See "Cheng wu" 程寤 in Li Xueqin 2010–2016, vol. 1, 下, 136.

38. See the studies in Cook and Major 1999.

39. See Da Haobo 2011; for the Shang evidence of relations with this region, see Shen Jianhua 2013.

40. *Zuozhuan*, Xiang 9 in *Chunqiu Zuozhuan zhengyi* 30.1941; for an attempt to trace Ji Lian and Yu Xiong's movements, see Li Yuhao 2013.

41. Shu Yi bells, *Jicheng* 272, 85.

42. After Buddhism spread to China, there were many accounts of Buddha's birth out of his mother's side in the Buddhist scriptures dating after the Han. For example, "Indra personally said that 'I am come from a split but a spacious place!' 'When Pusa first came down, s/he transformed into a white elephant crowned with a halo, the mother went into her bedroom during the day and had a dream about it (the birth). Something entered her right side while she slept and dreamed. . . . until the night of the eighth day of the fourth month when the stars came out, it transformed, being born out of her right side, dropped to the ground, and walked seven steps." See "Taizi Ruiyin benqi jing" 太子瑞應本起經, *Da zheng xinxiu Dazang jing*, vol. 3, 185; Rao Zongyi 1997, 16. The Indo-European "split birth" tales emerge also in Greek and Roman mythology with Athena born out to Zeus's head and Caesar being cut out of his mother's body. We know of no scholarship that has attempted to trace the movement of this tale over time and geography, if indeed they are even related.

43. The birth of a splitting side was discussed by Rao Zongyi (1997, 24): "Lu Zhong's wife was Nü Ku of the Guifang people, who later bore the lineage name of Kui. Nü Gui was (also written as) Nü Gui, belonging to the Red Di peoples of the Chunqiu period. The Han people understood the Guifang tribe to be the antecedents to the Ling Qiang. The Xia (progenitor) Yu rose up from the western Qiang. The tale of his mother giving birth to him through a split in her back is similar to that of Lu Zhong. It is difficult to pin down the time period of Yu and Lu Zhong but both (tales) derived from the Western Qiang, so the split-side birthing tale started with the Qiang Rong and later spread to the Central Xia region."

Conclusion

1. See "Gaozu benji" 高祖本紀, *Shiji* (Takikawa 1977, 8.4).

Bibliography

Ai Lan 艾蘭. *Gui zhi mi—Shang dai shenhua, jisi, yishu he yuzhouguan yanjiu* 龜之謎—商代神話、祭祀、藝術和宇宙觀研究. Revised. Beijing: Shangwu, 2010.
Ai Lan, and Wei Kebin 魏克彬, eds. *Guodian Laozi—dongxifang xuezhe de Duihua* 郭店老子——東西方學者的對話. Trans. Xing Wen 邢文. Beijing: Xueyuan, 2002.
Allan, S. *The Shape of the Turtle: Myth, Art, and Cosmos in Early China*. Albany: State University of New York Press, 1991.
Allan, S. *The Way of Water and Sprouts of Virtue*. Albany: State University of New York Press, 1997.
Allan, S. "The Great One, Water, and the *Laozi*: New Light from Guodian." *T'oung Pao* 89 (2003): 237–285.
Allan, S. "On the Identity of Shangdi 上帝 and the Origin of the Concept of a Celestial Mandate (*tian ming* 天命)." *Early China* 31 (2007): 1–46.
Allan, S. "Not the *lun yu*: The Chu Script Bamboo Slip Manuscript, *Zigao*, and the Nature of Early Confucianism." *Bulletin of the School of Oriental and African Studies* 72.1 (2009): 115–151.
Allan, S. "He Flies Like a Bird; He Dives Like a Dragon; Who Is That Man in the Tiger Mouth? Shamanic Images in Shang and Early Western Zhou Art." *Orientations* 41.3 (April 2010): 45–51.
Allan, S. "'When Red Pigeons Gathered on Tang's House': A Warring States Period Tale of Shamanic Possession and Building Construction Set at the Turn of the Xia and Shang Dynasties." *Journal of the Royal Asiatic Society* (April 2015): 1–20.
Allan, S. *Buried Ideas: Legends of Abdication and Ideal Government in Early Chinese Bamboo-Slip Manuscripts*. Albany: State University of New York Press, 2015.
Bai Yulan 白於藍. "Shi Xuanjiu" 釋玄咎. www.jianbo.org. Jianbo yanjiuwang, 1/19/2003.
Baxter, W. H., and L. Sagart. *Old Chinese: A New Reconstruction*. Oxford: Oxford University Press, 2014.
Brashier, K. E. *Ancestral Memory in Early China*. Cambridge: Harvard University Asia Center, 2011.

Bray, F. *Technology and Gender: Fabrics of Power in Late Imperial China*. Berkeley: University of California Press, 1997.

Cahill, S. *Transcendence and Divine Passion: The Queen Mother of the West in Medieval China*. Palo Alto: Stanford University Press, 1993.

Cai Wei 蔡偉. "Shi 'shen sheng'" 釋'慎聖.'" Fudan daxue chutu wenxian yu guwenzi yanjiu zhongxin. http://www.gwz.fudan.edu.cn, /5/23/2009. Accessed 2/26/2017.

Cai Yunzhang 蔡運章. "Lun Qin jian 'Bi' gua de yuzhou shengcheng moshi" 論秦簡《比》卦的宇宙生成模式. *Henan keji daxue xuebao* 4 (2004): 11–14.

Cai Yunzhang. "Qin jian 'Gua,' 'Tian,' 'X' zhugua jiegu—jian lun 'Guicang Yi' de ruogan wenti" 秦簡《寡》、《天》、《X》諸卦解詁—兼論《歸藏易》的若干問題. *Zhongyuan wenwu* 1 (2005): 42–52, 68.

Cao Feng 曹峰. "*Laozi* shouzhang yu 'ming' xiangguan wenti de chongxin shenshi" 《老子》首章與 "名" 相關問題的重新審視. *Zhexue yanjiu* 4 (2011): 58–67.

Cao Zhaolan 曹兆蘭. *Jinwen yu Yin Zhou nüxing wenhua* 金文與殷周女性文化. Beijing: Beijing University Press, 2004.

Chen Huan 陳奐 (1786–1863). *Maoshi zhuanshu* 毛詩傳疏. Ed. Wang Xianqian. *Qing jingjie xubian* 清經解續編. Vol. 3. Shanghai: Shanghai shudian, 1988.

Chen Jian 陳劍. "Shuo shen" 說慎. *Jianbo yanjiu* 簡帛研究二〇〇一. 1 (2001): 207–214.

Chen Jian. "Shangbo jian 'Zi Gao,' 'Cong zheng' pian de pinhe yu bianlian wenti xiaoyi" 上博簡《子羔》《從政》篇的拼合與編連問題小議. *Wenwu* 5 (2003): 56–59, 64.

Chen Mengjia 陳夢家. "Gaomei jiaoshe zumiao tongkao" 高禖郊社祖廟通考. *Qinghua daxue xuebao* 3 (1937): 445–472.

Chen Mengjia. "Cai qi san ji" 蔡器三記. *Kaogu* 7 (1963): 381–84, 361.

Chen Mengjia. *Yinxu buci zongshu* 殷虛卜辭綜述. Beijing: Zhonghua shuju, 1988.

Chen Minzhen 陳民鎮. "Du Qinghua jian *Chu ju* zhaji (er ze)" 讀清華簡《楚居》札記 (二則). http//:www.gwx.fudan.edu.cn, 5/31/2011. Accessed 2/26/2017.

Chen Songchang 陳松長, ed. *Xianggang Zhongwen daxue guan cang jiandu* 香港中文大學文物館藏簡牘. Hong Kong: Chinese University of Hong Kong Press, 2001.

Chen Shouqi 陳壽祺 (1771–1834). *Wujing yiyi shuzheng* 五經異義疏證. Ed. Ruan Yuan. *Qing jingjie* 清經解. Shanghai: Shanghai, 1988. Folio 7.

Chen Qiyou 陳奇猷, ed. *Lüshi chunqiu xin jiaoshi* 呂氏春秋新校釋. Shanghai: Guji, 2002.

Chen Wei 陳偉. *Baoshan Chu jian chutan* 包山楚簡初探. Wuhan: Wuhan University Press, 1996.

Chen Wei. "Chu ren daoci jilu zhong de rengui xitong yiji xiangguan wenti" 楚人禱祠記錄中的人鬼系統以及相關問題. 7/2/2008. http://www.bsm.org.cn/show_article.php?id=788. Accessed 3/17/2015.

Chen Wei. "Qinghua jian *Chu ju* 'pian shi' gushi xiaokao 清華簡《楚居》"梗室" 故事小考. http://www.bsm.org.cn/show_article.php?id=1398#. 2/3/2011. Accessed 2/26/2017.

Chen Yingjie 陳英傑. *Xi Zhou jinwen zuoqi yongtu mingci yanjiu* 西周金文作器用途銘辭研究. 2 Vols. Beijing: Xianzhuang, 2008.
Chen Zhi 陳致, ed. *Jianbo. Jingdian. Gushi* 簡帛·經典·古史. Shanghai: Shanghai guji, 2013.
Childs-Johnson, E. "Excavation of Tomb No. 5 at Yinxu, Anyang." *Chinese Sociology and Anthropology* 15.3 (Spring 1983).
Childs-Johnson, E. "The Bird in Shang Ritual Art: Intermediary to the Supernatural." *Orientations* (November 1989): 53–60.
Childs-Johnson, E. "The Metamorphic Image: A Predominant Theme in the Ritual Art of Shang China." *Bulletin of the Museum of Far Eastern Antiquities* 70 (1998): 5–171.
Childs-Johnson, E. "Jade as Confucian Ideal, Immortal Cloak, and Medium for the Metamorphic 'Fetal Pose.'" In *Enduring Art of Jade Age China, Vol. II: Chinese Jades of Late Neolithic Through Han Periods*, ed. E. Childs-Johnson, 15–24. New York: Throckmorton Fine Art, 2002.
Childs-Johnson, E. *The Meaning of the Graph Yi and Its Implications for Shang Belief and Art*. East Asia Journal Monograph No. 1. London: Saffron, 2008.
Chow Tse-tsung. "The Childbirth Myth and Ancient Chinese Medicine: A Study of Aspects of the *wu* Tradition." In *Ancient China: Studies in Early Civilization*, ed. D. T. Roy and T. Tsien. 43–89. Hong Kong: Chinese University of Hong Kong Press, 1978.
Chuci buzhu 楚辭補注. See Hong Xingzu, ed.
Chunqiu Zuozhuan zhengyi. See Kong Yingda, ed.
Cook, C. A. "Auspicious Metals and Southern Spirits: An Analysis of the Chu Bronze Inscriptions." University of California, Berkeley, PhD dissertation, 1990.
Cook, C. A. "Three High Gods of Chu." *Journal of Chinese Religions* 12 (1994): 1–23.
Cook, C. A. "Moonshine and Millet: Feasting and Purification Rituals in Ancient China." In *Of Tripod and Palate: Food, Politics, and Religion in Traditional China*, ed. R. Sterckx, 9–33. New York: Palgrave Macmillan, 2005.
Cook, C. A. *Death in Ancient China: The Tale of One Man's Journey*. Leiden: Brill, 2006.
Cook, C. A. "Ancestor Worship during the Eastern Zhou." In *Early Chinese Religion, Part One: Shang through Han (1250 BC–220 AD)*, vol. 1, ed. J. Lagerwey and M. Kalinowski, 237–279. Leiden: Brill, 2009.
Cook, C. A. "The Sage King Yu 禹 and the Bin Gong *xu* 豳公盨." *Early China* 35 (2012–2013): 69–103.
Cook, C. A. *Ancestors, Kings, and the Dao*. Cambridge: Harvard Asia Publications, 2017.
Cook, C. A., and J. S. Major, eds. *Defining Chu: Image and Reality in Ancient China*. Honolulu: University of Hawai'i Press, 1999.
Cook, C. A., and Zhao Lu. *Stalk Divination: A Newly Discovered Alternative to the "I Ching."* Oxford: Oxford University Press, 2017.

Cook, S. *The Bamboo Texts of Guodian: A Study and Complete Translation*. Cornell East Asia Series 164. 2 vols. Ithaca: Cornell University Press, 2012.
Da Dai Liji jinzhu jinyi 大戴禮記今註今譯, ed. Gao Ming 高明. Taipei: Taiwan Shangwu, 1993. 3rd rpt.
Da Haobo 笪浩波. "Cong jinnian chutu wenxian kan zaoqi Chu guo zhongxin quyu" 從近年出土文獻看早期楚國中心區域. http://www.gwz.Fudan.edu.cn/, 6/2/11. Accessed 2/26/2017.
Da zheng xinxiu Dazang jing 大正新修大藏經. Vol. 3, 185. "Taizi Ruiyin benqi jing" 太子瑞應本起經. http://www.cbeta.org/result/normal/T03/0185_001.htm. Accessed 2/26/2017.
Dai Nianzu 戴念祖. "Shixi Qin jian *Lüshu* zhong de yuelü yu zhanbu" 試析秦簡《律書》中的樂律與占卜. *Zhongguo yinyuexue* 2 (2001): 5–10.
Demattè, P. "Antler and Tongue: New Archaeological Evidence in the Study of Chu Tomb Guardian." *East and West* 44.2–4 (December 1994): 353–404.
Deng Peiling 鄧佩玲. *Tianming, guishen yu zhudao—Dong Zhou jinwen jiaci tanlun* 天命、鬼神與祝禱——東周金文嘏辭探論. Taipei: Yiwen, 2011.
Despeux, C., and L. Kohn. *Women in Daoism*. Cambridge: Three Pines Press, 2003.
Dexter, M. R., and V. Mair. *Sacred Display: Divine and Magical Female Figures of Eurasia*. Amherst: Cambria, 2010.
Ding Sixin 丁四新. *Guodian Chu zhushu* Laozi *jiaozhu* 郭店楚竹書《老子》校注. Wuhan: Wuhan daxue, 2010.
Ding Sixin, ed. *Chu zhushu yu Han boshu* Zhouyi *jiaozhu* 楚竹書與漢帛書《周易》校注. Shanghai: Shanghai guji, 2011.
Du Lanfang 杜蘭芳 and Gu Jianghong 顧江紅. "Gudai yiji zhong dui nanchan de miaoshu" 古代醫籍中對難產的描述. *Xibu Zhong yiyao* 25.2 (2012): 47–49.
Duan Yucai 段玉裁. *Shuowen jiezi zhu* 說文解字注 Shanghai: Shanghai guji, 1988.
Erya zhushu. See Kong Yingda, ed.
Falkenhausen, L. "The Waning of the Bronze Age: Material Culture and Social Developments, 770–481 B.C." In *The Cambridge History of Ancient China: From the Origins of Civilization to 221 B.C.*, ed. M. Loewe and E. L. Shaughnessy, 450–544. Cambridge: Cambridge University Press, 1999.
Falkenhausen, L. *Chinese Society in the Age of Confucius (1000–250 BC): The Archaeological Evidence*. Los Angeles: Cotsen Institute of Archaeology, University of California Press, 2006.
Fan Ye 范曄 (398–445) and Li Xian 李賢 (651–684), eds. *Houhanshu* 後漢書. Beijing: Zhonghua, 1965.
Fudan University Excavated Text and Paleographical Research Center Graduate Reading Group 復旦大學出土文獻與古文字研究中心研究生讀書會. "Qinghua jian *Chu ju* yandu zhaji" 清華簡《楚居》研讀札記. http://www.jianbo.org, 3/13/2011; http://www.gwz.fudan.edu.cn/, 5/1/2011. Accessed 2/26/2017.
Furth, C. *A Flourishing Yin: Gender in China's Medical History, 960–1665*. Berkeley: University of California Press, 1999.
Gansusheng wenwu kaogu yanjiusuo 甘肅省文物考古研究所. *Tianshui Fangmatan Qin jian* 天水放馬灘秦簡. Beijing: Zhonghua, 2009.

Gao Chongwen 高崇文. "Qinghua jian *Chu ju* suo zai Chu zaoqi judi bianxi" 清華簡《楚居》所載楚早期居地辨析. *Jianghan kaogu* 4 (2011): 61–67.

Goldin, P. R. "The View of Women in Early Confucianism." In *The Sage and the Second Sex: Confucianism, Ethics, and Gender*, ed. Chenyang Li, 133–161. Chicago and La Salle: Open Court, 2000.

Goldin, P. R. *The Culture of Sex in Ancient China*. Honolulu: University of Hawai'i Press, 2002.

Granet, M. *Fête et Chansons aciennes de la Chine*. Paris: Albin Michel, 1919. Rpt. 1982.

Granet, M. *Danses et legends de la Chine ancienne*. 2 Vols. Paris: Universitaires de France, 1926. Rpt. Editions d'aujourd'hui, 1982.

Guo Moruo 郭沫若. *Liangzhou jinwenci daxi tulu kaoshi* 兩周金文辭大系圖錄考釋. Shanghai: Shanghai shudian, 1999.

Guo Moruo. *Guo Moruo quanji* 郭沫若全集. Beijing: Kexue, 1982.

Guo Moruo, Hu Houxuan 胡厚宣, et al., eds. *Jiaguwen heji* 甲骨文合集. 13 Vols. Beijing: Zhonghua, 1978–1982.

Guo Ruoyu 郭若愚. "Cong you guan Cai Hou de ruogan ziliao lun Shouxian Cai Hou mu Cai qi de niandai" 從有關蔡侯的若干資料論壽縣蔡墓蔡器的年代. *Shanghai Bowuguan jikan* 2 (1982): 75–88.

Hall, D. L., and R. T. Ames. "Sexism, with Chinese Characteristics." In *The Sage and the Second Sex: Confucianism, Ethics, and Gender*, ed. Chenyang Li, 75–95. Chicago and La Salle: Open Court, 2000.

Hanshu 漢書. Beijing: Zhonghua, 1962.

Harper, D. "Demonography." *Harvard Journal of Asiatic Studies* 45.2 (1985): 459–498.

Harper, D. "The Sexual Arts of Ancient China as Described in a Manuscript of the Second Century B.C." *Harvard Journal of Asiatic Studies* 47.2 (1987): 539–593.

Harper, D. *Early Chinese Medical Literature: The Mawangdui Medical Manuscripts*. London: Kegan Paul In ternational, 1998.

Harper, D. "Warring States Natural Philosophy and Occult Thought." In *The Cambridge History of Ancient China: From the Origins of Civilization to 221 B.C.*, ed. M. Loewe and E. L. Shaughnessy, 813–884. Cambridge: Cambridge University Press, 1999.

Harper, D. "The Nature of Taiyi in the Guodian Manuscript *Taiyi sheng shui*: Abstract Cosmic Principle or Supreme Cosmic Deity?" *Chūgoku shutsudo shiryō kenkyū* 中國出土資料研究 5 (2001): 1–23.

Harper, D. "Spellbinding." In *Religions of Asia in Practice: An Anthology*, ed. D. S. Lopez, 376–385. Princeton: Princeton University Press, 2002.

Harper, D., and M. Kalinowski, eds. *Books of Fate and Popular Culture in Early China: The Daybook Manuscripts of the Warring States, Qin, and Han*. Leiden: Brill, forthcoming.

Hawkes, D. *The Songs of the South: An Anthology of Ancient Chinese Poems by Qu Yuan and Other Poets*. Middlesex: Penguin, 1985.

He Xin 何新. *Yuzhou de qiyuan: Chu boshu yu Xia xiaozheng xinkao* 宇宙的起源: 《楚帛書》與《夏小正》新考. Beijing: Zhongguo minzhu fazhi, 2008.

He Yaohua 何耀華. "Yi zu de ziran chongbai ji qi tedian" 彝族的自然崇拜及其特点. *Sixiang zhanxian* 思想戰線6 (1982): 69–79.

Hebu. See Peng Bangjiong et al.

Heji. See Guo Moruo et al.

Henansheng wenwu kaogu suo 河南省文物考古所, ed. *Xin Cai Geling Chu mu* 新蔡葛陵楚墓. Zhengzhou: Daxiang, 2003.

Henricks, R. G. *Lao Tzu's Tao Te Ching: A Translation of the Startling New Documents Found at Guodian.* Translations from the Asian Classics. New York: Columbia University Press, 2000.

Hinrichs, T. J., and L. L. Barnes, eds. *Chinese Medicine and Healing: An Illustrated History.* Cambridge: Belknap Press, 2013.

Hong Xingzu 洪興祖 (1090–1155) (with index by Takeji Sadao 竹治貞夫), ed. *Chuci buzhu fu suoyin* 楚辭補注附索引. Taipei: Zhongwen, 1979.

Hou Han shu. See Fan Ye and Li Xian.

Hu Houxuan 胡厚宣. "Chu minzu yuanyu dongfangkao" 楚民族源於東方考. *Shixue luncong* 史學論叢. Vol. 1. Beijing: Beijing daxue qianshe 北京大學潛社, 1934. Chapter 7.

Hu Houxuan. "Yindai hunyin jiazu zongfa shengyu zhidu kao" 殷代婚姻家族宗法生育制度考. *Chengdu Qi Lu daxue guoxue yanjiusuo congkan* 成都齊魯大學國學研究所叢刊1944. Rpt. *Jiaguxue shangshi luncong chuji (waiyizhong) shang, xia* 甲骨學商史論叢初集 (外一種) 上、下. Shijiazhuang: Hebei jiaoyu, 2002. 82–133.

Huainanzi. See Liu Wendian 劉文典.

Huang Guangwu 黃光武. "Jinwen zisun chengwei chongwen de shidu ji qifa" 金文子孫稱謂重文的釋讀及啟發. *Zhongshan daxue xuebao* 中山大學學報4 (1992): 124–126.

Huang Guohui 黃國輝. "Shangdai qincheng qubiezi ruogan wenti yanjiu" 商代親稱區別字若干問題研究. *Kaogu xuebao* 3 (2012): 262–288. Rpt. in *Xian Qin, Qin Han shi* 6 (2012): 3–15.

Huang Xiquan 黃錫全. "Chu jian zhong de X Yin X Yin yu X Yin Xue Yin zaiyi" 楚簡中的XX與XX再議. *Jianbo yanjiu* 2004 (2006): 7–12.

Huangfu Mi 皇甫謐, comp. *Di wang shiji* 帝王世紀. Jinan: Qi Lu, 1998.

Hubeisheng bowuguan 湖北省博物館. *Zeng Hou Yi mu* 曾侯乙墓. Beijing: Wenwu, 1989.

Hubeisheng bowuguan, ed. *Zeng Hou Yi mu wenwu yishu* 曾侯乙墓文物藝術. Wuhan: Hubei meishu, 1991.

Institute of History and Philology, Academia Sinica 中央研究院歷史語言研究所. *Digital Archive of Bronze Images and Inscriptions* 殷周金文暨青銅器資料庫. http://www.ihp.sinica.edu.tw/~bronze/, 2009. Accessed 2/26/2017.

Jia, Jinhua, Xiaofei Kang, and Ping Yao, eds. *Gendering Chinese Religion: Subject, Identity, and Body.* Albany: State University of New York Press, 2014.

Jia Wen 賈文. "Shuo 'ming'" 說 '冥.' *Yindu xuekan* 1 (1996). Rpt. in *Jiaguwenxian jicheng: jiaguexue tonglun* 甲骨文獻集成: 甲骨學通論, ed. Song Zhenhao 宋鎮豪, Duan Zhihong 段志洪, Chen Jianhua 陳建華, Cai Zhongmin 蔡忠民, and Tang Defeng 唐德風, vol. 14, 176–177. Chengdu: Sichuan daxue, 2001.

Jiaguwen heji. See Guo Moruo et al.

Jiang Linchang 江林昌 and Sun Jin 孫進. "*Chu ju* 'xiesheng' 'bintian' de shenhuaxue yu kaoguxue yanjiu" 《楚居》"胥生" "賓天" 的神話學與考古學研究. *Qinghua jian yanjiu* 1 (2012): 295–302.

Jicheng. See Zhongguo shehui kexueyuan kaogu yanjiusuo, comp.

Jin Xinzhou 金信周. "Liang Zhou zhujiaci mingwen yanjiu" 兩周頌揚銘文及其文化研究. Fudan University, PhD dissertation, 2006.

Kalinowski, M. "The *Xingde* 刑德 Texts from Mawangdui." *Early China* 23–24 (1998–1999): 126–202.

Ke Heli 柯鶴立. "Chu xianzu de dansheng gushi" 楚先祖的誕生故事. *Xian Qin shi yanjiu dongtai* 先秦史研究動態 2 (2013) 28–45. Revised version in *Chu jian Chu wenhua yu xian Qin lishi wenhua guoji xueshu yantaohui lunwenji* 楚簡楚文化與先秦歷史文化國際學術研討會論文集, ed. Luo Yunhuan, 134–155. Wuhan: Hubei jiaoyu, 2013.

Ke Heli 柯鶴立. "Shiyong Qinghuajian 'Shifa' jiedu Baoshan zhanbu jilu zhong gua yi" 試用清華簡《筮法》解讀包山占卜記錄中卦義. *Jianbo yanjiu* (2016): 12–22.

Keightley, D. N. "At the Beginning: The Status of Women in Neolithic and Shang China." *Nan nü: Men, Women and Gender in Early and Imperial China* 1.1 (1999): 1–63.

Keightley, D. N. *Working for His Majesty: Research Notes on Labor Mobilization in Late Shang China (ca. 1200–1045 B.C.), as Seen in the Oracle-Bone Inscriptions, with Particular Attention to Handicraft Industries, Agriculture, Warfare, Hunting, Construction, and the Shang's Legacies*. Institute of East Asian Studies China Research Monograph 67. Berkeley: University of California Press, 2012.

Kinney, A. *Representations of Childhood and Youth in Early China*. Palo Alto: Stanford University Press, 2004.

Knoblock, J. *Xunzi: A Translation and Study of the Complete Works*, vol. 3 (books 17–32). Stanford: Stanford University Press, 1994.

Kong Yingda 孔穎達 (574–648), ed. *Chunqiu Zuozhuan zhengyi* 春秋左傳正義. In *Shisanjing zhushu* vol. 2, ed. Ruan Yuan. Beijing: Zhonghua, 1980. Rpt. 2008.

Kong Yingda, ed. *Liji zhengyi* 禮記正義. In *Shisanjing zhushu*, vol. 1, ed. Ruan Yuan. Beijing: Zhonghua, 1980.

Kong Yingda, ed. *Mao shi zhengyi* 毛詩正義. In *Shisanjing zhushu*, vol. 1, ed. Ruan Yuan. Beijing: Zhonghua, 1980.

Kong Yingda, ed. *Shangshu zhengyi* 尚書正義. In *Shisanjing zhushu*, vol. 1, ed. Ruan Yuan. Beijing: Zhonghua, 1980.

Kong Yingda, ed. *Yili zhengyi* 儀禮正義. In *Shisanjing zhushu*, vol. 1, ed. Ruan Yuan. Beijing: Zhonghua, 1980.

Lagerwey, J., and M. Kalinowski, eds. *Early Chinese Religion, Part One: Shang through Han (1250 BC–220 AD)*. 2 vols. Leiden: Brill, 2009.

Lai, G. *Excavating the Afterlife: The Archaeology of Early Chinese Religion*. Seattle: University of Washington Press, 2015.

Lai, K. "The *Daodejing*: Resources for Contemporary Feminist Thinking." *Journal of Chinese Philosophy* 27.2 (2000): 131–153.

Lau, U., and T. Staack. *Legal Practice in the Formative Stages of the Chinese Empire: An Annotated Translation of the Exemplary Qin Criminal Cases from the Yuelu Academy Collection*. Leiden: Brill, 2016.

Lei Xueqi 雷學淇, ed. *Shiben bazhong* 世本八種. Shanghai: Shangwu, 1957.

Leung, A., ed. *Medicine for Women in Imperial China*. Leiden: Brill, 2006.

Lewis, M. E. *Sanctioned Violence in Early China*. Albany: State University of New York Press, 1990.

Lewis, M. E. *The Construction of Space in Early China*. Albany: State University of New York Press, 2006a.

Lewis, M. E. *The Flood Myths of Early China*. Albany: State University of New York Press, 2006b.

Li Binghai 李炳海. "Xian Qin liang Han sanwen de mengxiang yu shengzhi chongbai" 先秦兩漢散文的夢象與生殖崇拜. *Xueshu jiaoliu* 160.7 (2007): 138–141.

Li, C., ed. *The Sage and the Second Sex*. Chicago: Open Court, 2000.

Li, F. *Bureaucracy and the State in Early China: Governing the Western Zhou*. Cambridge: Cambridge University Press, 2008.

Li Fengxiang 黎鳳翔, ed. *Guanzi jiaozhu* 管子校注. Beijing: Zhonghua, 2004.

Li Hong 李虹. "*Shijing* zhong 'caiji yu hunlian' zhuti yanjiu" 《詩經》中'采集與婚戀' 主題研究. *Shaanxi shifan daxue xuebao* 30 (2001): 241–244.

Li Jiahao 李家浩. "Chu jian suo ji Chu ren zuxian 'X (yu) Xiong' yu 'Xue Xiong' wei yi ren shuo" 楚簡所記楚人祖先 "X (鬻) 熊" 與 "穴熊" 為一人說. *Wenshi* 3 (2010): 5–44.

Li Jiahao. "Tan Qinghua Zhanguo zhujian *Chu ju* de 'Yitun' ji qita—jian tan Baoshan Chu jian de 'Tun ren' deng" 談清華戰國竹簡《楚居》的 "夷X" 及其他——兼談包山楚簡的 "X 人" 等. *Qinghua jian yanjiu* 1 (2012): 248–260.

Li Ling 李零. *Changsha Zidanku Zhanguo Chu boshu yanjiu* 長沙子彈庫楚帛書研究. Beijing: Zhonghua, 1985.

Li Ling. "Kaogu faxian yu shenhua chuanshuo" 考古發現與神話傳說. *Xueren* 學人 5 (1994): 115–150.

Li Ling. "Du Qinghua jian biji: X yu Qie" 讀清華簡筆記: X 與竊. *Qinghua jian yanjiu* 1 (2012): 330–334.

Li Min 李民. *Yin shang shehui shenghuo shi* 殷商社會生活史. Zhengzhou: Henan renmin, 1993.

Li Shoukui 李守奎. "Lun *Chu ju* zhong Ji Lian yu Yu Xiong shiji de chuanshuo tezheng" 論《楚居》中季連與鬻熊事迹的傳說特征. *Qinghua daxue xuebao* 26

(2011) 4: 33–39. Rpt. in *Gudai jiandu baohu yu zhengli yanjiu* 古代簡牘保護文獻與整理研究, ed. Qinghua daxue chutu wenxian yanjiu yu baohu zhongxin 清華大學出土文獻研究與保護中心, Beijing daxue chutu wenxian yanjiusuo 北京大學出土文獻研究所, Jingzhou wenwu baohu zhongxin 荊州文物保護中心, 191–200. Shanghai: Zhongxi, 2012.

Li Shoukui. "Genju *Chu ju* jiedu shishu zhong Xiong Qu zhi Xiong Yan shixu zhi hunluan 根據《楚居》解讀史書中熊渠至熊延世序之混亂. In *Gudai jiandu baohu yu zhengli yanjiu*, ed. Qinghua daxue chutu wenxian yanjiu yu baohu zhongxin, Beijing daxue chutu wenxian yanjiusuo, Jingzhou wenwu baohu zhongxin, 201–208. Shanghai: Zhongxi, 2012.

Li Shoukui, Qu bing 曲冰, Sun Weilong 孫偉龍, eds. "Fulu 6, Shiwen" 附錄 6, 釋文. *Shanghai bowuguan cang Zhanguo Chu zhushu (1–5) wenzi bian* 上海博物館藏戰國楚竹書（一–五）文字編. Beijing: Zuojia, 2007. 802.

Li Jia 李佳. "Shengzhi zhi zhudao, hunpin zhi xinwu—*Shijing* zhong lu yixiang de xiangzheng jieyi" 生殖之祝禱，婚聘之信物——《詩經》中鹿意象的象徵性解疑. *Hebei shifan daxue xuebao* 35.3 (2012): 72–77.

Li Xueqin 李學勤. "Lun Baoshan jian zhong yi Chu xianzu ming" 論包山簡中一楚先祖名. *Wenwu* 8 (1988): 87–88.

Li Xueqin. "Qinghua jian jiupian zongshu" 清華簡九篇綜述. *Wenwu* 5 (2010): 50–57.

Li Xueqin. "Lun Qinghua jian *Chu ju* zhong de gushi chuanshuo" 論清華簡《楚居》中的古史傳說. *Zhongguo shi yanjiu* 1 (2011). Rpt. in *Gudai jiandu baohu yu zhengli yanjiu* 古代簡牘保護文獻與整理研究, ed. Qinghua daxue chutu wenxian yanjiu yu baohu zhongxin 清華大學出土文獻研究與保護中心, Beijing daxue chutu wenxian yanjiusuo 北京大學出土文獻研究所, Jingzhou wenwu baohu zhongxin 荊州文物保護中心, 162–168. Shanghai: Zhongxi, 2012.

Li Xueqin. "Qinghua jian *Chu ju* yu Chu xi Xunying" 清華簡《楚居》與楚徙鄩郢. Rpt. *Gudai jiandu baohu yu zhengli yanjiu* 古代簡牘保護文獻與整理研究, ed. Qinghua daxue chutu wenxian yanjiu yu baohu zhongxin 清華大學出土文獻研究與保護中心, Beijing daxue chutu wenxian yanjiusuo 北京大學出土文獻研究所, Jingzhou wenwu baohu zhongxin 荊州文物保護中心, 269–171. Shanghai: Zhongxi, 2012.

Liu Xiang 刘翔 Chen Kang 陈抗 Chen Chusheng 陈初生, Dong Kun 董琨 Li Xueqin, ed. *Shang Zhou guwenzi duben* 商周古文字讀本. Beijing: Yuwen, 1989.

Li Xueqin, ed. *Qinghua daxue cang Zhanguo zhujian* 清華大學藏戰國竹簡. 6 Vols. Shanghai: Wenyi, 2010–2016.

Li Yuhao 李玉浩. "*Chu ju* jizai de Ji Lian zhi Yu Xiong qianxi yu huodong diyu kaoshu" 《楚居》記載的季連至鬻熊遷徙與活動地域考述. Luo Yunhuan, ed. (2013): 204–211.

Liang Qing 梁晴 and Xue Xiuying 薛秀英. "Jianlun jiaguwen zhong guanyu shengyu de wenti" 简论甲骨文中关于生育的问题. *Zhongyuan wenwu* 3 (1986): 92–93. Rpt. in *Jiaguwenxian jicheng: jiaguexue tonglun* 甲骨文獻集

成: 甲骨學通論, ed. Song Zhenhao 宋鎮豪, Duan Zhihong 段志洪, Chen Jianhua 陳建華, Cai Zhongmin 蔡忠民, and Tang Defeng 唐德風, vol. 29, 313. Chengdu: Sichuan daxue, 2001.

Lin Zhongjun 林忠軍. "Qinghua jia Shifa shizhanfa tanwei" 清華簡《筮法》筮占法探微. Zhongguo shehui kexue wang. 9/29/2014. http://phil.cssn.cn/zhx/zx_zgzx/201409/t20140929_1347214_3.shtml. Accessed 2/27/2015.

Liji zhengyi 禮記正義. See Ruan Yuan 1980, vol. 2.

Liu Hehui 劉和惠. "Cai qi mingyu Chu Cai guanxi xintan" 蔡器銘與楚蔡關係新探. Dongnan wenhua 東南文化 3 (1989): 22–28.

Liu Huan 劉桓. "Yinxu buci zhong de 'duoyu' wenti" 殷墟卜辭中的 '多毓' 問題. Kaogu 5 (2010): 61–68.

Liu Lexian 劉樂賢. Shuihudi Qin jian rishu yanjiu 睡虎地秦簡日書研究. Dalu diqu boshi lunwen series 大陸地區博士論文叢刊. Taipei: Wenjian, 1993.

Liu Lexian. "Shuihudi Qin jian rishu 'renzi pian' yanjiu" 睡虎地秦簡 "人字篇" 研究. Jiang Han kaogu 1 (1995a): 58–61.

Liu Lexian. "Shuihudi Qin jian rishu 'renzi pian' bushi" 睡虎地秦簡 "人字篇" 補釋. Jiang Han kaogu 2 (1995b): 82–83.

Liu Lexian. Jianbo shushu wenxian tanlun 簡帛數術文獻探論. Beijing: Renmin daxue, 2012.

Liu Tao 劉濤. "Qinghua jian Chu ju zhong suo jian wufeng kao" 清華簡《楚居》中所見巫風考. www.gwz.fudan.edu.cn, 6/19/2011

Liu Tseng-kuei. "Taboos: An Aspect of Belief." In Early Chinese Religion, Part One: Shang through Han (1250 BC–220 AD), ed. J. Lagerwey and M. Kalinowski, vol. 2, 881–948. Leiden: Brill, 2009.

Liu Wendian 劉文典 (1893–1958). Huainan honglie jijie 淮南鴻烈集解. Beijing: Zhonghua, 1989.

Liu Xiang, ed. Shang Zhou guwenzi duben 商周古文字讀本. Beijing: Yuwen, 1989.

Liu Xiaogan 劉笑敢. "Guanyu Laozi zhi cixing biyu de quanshi wenti" 關於《老子》之雌性比喻的詮釋問題. Zhongguo wenzhe yanjiu jikan 23 (2003): 179–209.

Liu Xiaogan. Laozi gujin: wuzhong duikan yu xiping yinlun 老子古今: 五種對勘與析評引論. Revised ed. Beijing: Zhongguo shehui kexue, 2006.

Liu Xinfang 劉信芳. "Chu boshu Fuxi Nüwa kao" 楚帛書伏羲女媧考. Jianbo yanjiu (2002–2003): 135–143.

Liu Xinfang. "Zhushu Chu ju 'wenqi,' 'xiechu,' 'Xiongda' de shidu yu shishi" 竹書《楚居》"問期"、"脅出"、"熊達" 的釋讀與史實. Jiang Han kaogu 1 (2013): 123–126.

Loewe, M., and E. L. Shaughnessy, eds. The Cambridge History of Ancient China: From the Origins of Civilization to 221 B.C. Cambridge: Cambridge University Press, 1999.

Lü Yahu 呂亞虎. "Boshu 'Taichan shu' suojian zaoqi yunyu xinyang qianxi" 帛書《胎產書》所見早期孕育信仰淺析. Jiang Han luntan 6 (2009): 70–77.

Lunheng zhushi 論衡注釋. Beijing: Zhonghua, 1979.

Luo Erhu 羅二虎. *Handai huaxiang shiguan* 漢代畫像石棺. Chengdu: Ba Shu, 2002.
Luo Xiaohua 羅小華. *Shi bin* 釋賓. *Jianbo* 5 (2010): 117–121.
Luo Xinhui 羅新慧. *Shouyangjijin shuzheng* 首陽吉金疏證. Shanghai: Shanghai guji, 2016.
Luo Yuankai 羅元愷. "Zhongguo fukexue de yuanliu he fazhan" 中國婦科學的源流和發展. *Guangzhou yixueyuan xuebao* 7.4 (1990): 197–203.
Luo Yunhuan 羅運環. "Guanyu Ji Lian jiuge wenti de tantao" 關於季連糾葛問題的探討. *Qinghua jian yanjiu* 1 (2012): 287–394.
Luo Yunhuan, ed. *Chu jian Chu wenhua yu xian Qin lishi wenhua guoji xueshu yantaohui lunwenji* 楚簡楚文化與先秦歷史文化國際學術研討會論文集. Wuhan: Hubei jiaoyu, 2013.
Ma, L. "Character of the Feminine in Levinas and the *Daodejing* 道德經." *Journal of Chinese Philosophy* 36.3 (2009): 261–276.
Ma, L. "Levinas and the *Daodejing* on the Feminine: Intercultural Reflections." *Journal of Chinese Philosophy* 39.1 (2012): 152–170.
Ma Chengyuan 馬承源, and Shanghai bowuguan, comp. *Shang Zhou qingtongqi mingwenxuan* 商周青銅器銘文選. 4 vols. Beijing: Wenwu, 1986–1988.
Ma Chengyuan, ed. *Shanghai bowuguan cang Zhanguo Chu zhushu* 上海博物館藏戰國楚竹書. 8 vols. Shanghai: Shanghai guji, 2001–2011.
Ma Jixing 馬繼興. *Mawangdui gu yishu kaoshi* 馬王堆古醫書考釋. Changsha: Hunan kejixue jishu, 1992.
Ma Ruichen 馬瑞辰 (1777–1853). *Maoshi zhuan jian tongshi 32 juan* 毛詩傳箋通釋32卷. Beijing: Zhonghua, 1989.
Major, J. S. "The Meaning of *Hsing-te*." In *Chinese Ideas about Nature and Society: Studies in Honour of Derk Bodde*, ed. C. le Blanc and S. Blader, 281–291. Hong Kong: University of Hong Kong Press, 1987.
Major, J. S., and C. A. Cook. *Ancient China: A History*. New York and London: Routledge, 2016.
Maoshi zhengyi. See Kong Yingda, ed.
Meng Pengsheng 孟蓬生. "*Chu ju* suojian Chu wangming kaoshi erze" 《楚居》所見楚王名考釋二則. *Qinghua jian yanjiu* 1 (2012): 303–312.
Mozi jiangu. See Sun Yirang, *Zhuzi jicheng*, vol. 4.
Niu Pengtao 牛鵬濤. "Shilun Qinghua jian *Chu ju* zhi gushi guan" 試論清華簡《楚居》之古史觀. In *Chu jian Chu wenhua yu xian Qin lishi wenhua guoji xueshu yantaohui lunwenji*, ed. Luo Yunhuan, 181–188. Wuhan: Hubei jiaoyu, 2013.
Pankenier, D. "A Brief History of the Beiji (Northern Culmen), with an Excursus on the Origin of the Character *di* 帝." *Journal of the American Oriental Society* 124.2 (2004): 211–236.
Peng Bangjiong 彭邦炯. "Jiaguwen zhong de shengyu wenti zai tansuo" 甲骨文中的生育問題再探索. *Yindu xuekan* 1 (2006): 5–9.
Peng Bangjiong, Xie Ji 謝濟, and Ma Jifan 馬季凡. *Jiaguwen heji bubian* 甲骨文合集補編. 7 vols. Beijing: Yuyan, 1999.

Pines, Y. "Disputers of Abdication: Zhanguo Egalitarianism and the Sovereign's Power." *T'oung Pao* 91 (2005): 243–300.
Poo, Mu-chou. *In Search of Personal Welfare: A View of Ancient Chinese Religion*. Albany: State University of New York Press, 1998.
Pu Maozuo 濮茅左. "Jiaguwen zhong suojian de you guan yunyuzi" 甲骨文中所見的有關孕育字. *Zhonghua yishi zazhi* 中華醫史雜志 1 (1985). Rpt. in *Jiaguwenxian jicheng: jiaguexue tonglun* 甲骨文獻集成: 甲骨學通論, ed. Song Zhenhao 宋鎮豪, Duan Zhihong 段志洪, Chen Jianhua 陳建華, Cai Zhongmin 蔡忠民, and Tang Defeng 唐德風, vol. 29, 307. Chengdu: Sichuan daxue, 2001.
Wenxin 齊文心 and Wang Guimin 王貴民. "Shang Xizhou wenhuazhi" 商西周文化志. *Lidai wenhu yange* series, vol. 1. Shanghai: Shanghai guji, 1998.
Qiao Anshui 喬安水. "Yinyang zhexue tanyuan" 陰陽哲學探源. *Yantai daxue xuebao* 16.3 (2003): 250–254.
Qinghua daxue chutu wenxian yanjiu yu baohu zhongxin 清華大學出土文獻研究與保護中心, Beijing daxue chutu wenxian yanjiusuo 北京大學出土文獻研究所, Jingzhou wenwu baohu zhongxin 荊州文物保護中心, eds. *Gudai jiandu baohu yu zhengli yanjiu* 古代簡牘保護文獻與整理研究. Shanghai: Zhongxi, 2012.
Qiu Xigui 裘錫圭. "Shi Yin buci zhong de X, Y deng zi 釋殷虛卜辭中的X、Y等字." *Di erjie guoji Zhongguo guwenzi xueshu taolunhui lunwenji* 第二屆國際中國古文字學研討會論文集. Hong Kong: Chinese University of Hong Kong Press, 1993. 73–94.
Qiu Xigui. "Lun Yin xu buci 'duo yu' zhi 'yu'" 論殷墟卜辭「多毓」之「毓」. *Zhongguo Shang wenhua guoji xueshu taolunhui lunwenji* 中國商文化國際學術討論會論文集. Beijing: Zhongguo dabaike quan shu, 1998. 450–458.
Qiu Xigui. *Zhongguo chutu wenxian shi jiang* 中國出土文獻十講. Shanghai: Fudan University Press, 2004.
Qiu Xigui. "Guanyu shangdai de zongzu zuzhi yu guizu he pingmin liangge jieji de chubu yanjiu" 關於商代的宗族組織與貴族和平民兩個階級的初步研究. *Qiu Xigui xueshu wenji* 裘錫圭學術文集. Vol. 5. Shanghai: Fudan University Press, 2012.
Qiu Xigui. "'Dong Huang Taiyi' yu 'Da X Fuxi'" "東皇太一" 與 "大X 伏羲." In *Jianbo. Jingdian. Gushi*, ed. Chen Zhi, 1–15. Shanghai: Shanghai guji, 2013.
Raphals, L. *Sharing the Light: Representations of Women and Virtue in Early China*. Albany: State University of New York Press, 1998.
Rao Zongyi 饒宗頤. "Zhongguo gudai 'xiesheng' de chuanshuo" 中國古代 "眘生" 的傳說. *Yanjing xuebao* (New Series) 3 (1997): 15–28.
Rao Zongyi and Zeng Xiantong 曾憲通. *Chu boshu* 楚帛書. Hong Kong: Zhonghua, 1985.
Raz, G. "Birthing the Self: Metaphor and Transformation in Medieval Daoism." In *Gendering Chinese Religion: Subject, Identity, and Body*, ed. Jinhua Jia, Xiaofei Kang, and Ping Yao, 183–200. Albany: State University of New York Press, 2014.

Ross, S. "Mythology as an Indicator of Cultural Change. Hunting and Agriculture as Reflected in North American Traditions." *Anthropos* 95.2(2000): 433–443.

Ruan Yuan 阮元 (1764–1849), ed. *Shisanjing zhushu* 十三經注疏. 2 vols. Beijing: Zhonghua, 1980. Rpt. 2008.

Rutt, R. *Zhouyi: The Book of Changes*. Durham East-Asia Series No. 1. Richmond: Curzon, 1996.

Seligman, A. B., R. P. Weller, M. J. Puett, B. Simon. *Ritual and Its Consequences: An Essay on the Limits of Sincerity*. Oxford: Oxford University Press, 2008.

Schaberg, D. *A Patterned Past: Form and Thought in Early Chinese Historiography*. Cambridge: Harvard University Asia Center, 2001.

Shan Zhouyao 單周堯. "Du Qinghua jian *Chu ju* 'kui zi xie chu' yu 'Wu Binggai qi xie yi Chu'" xiaoshi 讀清華簡《楚居》"潰自脅出" 與 "巫並賅亓脅以楚" 小識, *Chu Jian, Chu wenhua yu Xian Qin lishi wenhua yantaohui lunwenji*, vol. 1 (Wuhan 2011), 87–96. Rpt. in *Xian Qin shi yanjiu dongtai* 先秦史研究動態 2 (2013): 46–57, and in *Chu jian Chu wenhua yu xian Qin lishi wenhua guoji xueshu yantaohui lunwenji* 楚簡楚文化與先秦歷史文化國際學術研討會論文集, ed. Luo Yunhuan, 122–133. Wuhan: Hubei jiaoyu, 2013.

Shan Zhouyao. "Du Qinghua jian *Chu ju* 'Bing Si X xiang X Zhou sifang' xiaoshi" 讀清華簡《楚居》'秉鉑衛相罾胄四方' 小識. In *Jianbo. Jingdian. Gushi*, ed. Chen Zhi, 135–141. Shanghai: Shanghai guji, 2013.

Shandong daxue lishi wenhua xueyuan kaoguxi 山東大學歷史文化學院考古系. "Changqing Xianrentai wuhaomu fajue jianbao" 長清仙人臺五號墓發掘簡報. *Wenwu* 9 (1998): 18–30.

Shanghai Bowuguan, ed. *Shanghai bowuguan cang Zhanguo Chu zhushu* 上海博物館藏戰國楚竹书. Vol. 2. Shanghai: Shanghai guji, 2002.

Shangshu. See Ruan Yuan 1980, vol. 1.

Shanhaijing jianshu 山海經箋疏, ed. Hao Yixing 郝懿行. Taipei: Yiwen, 1974. See also Yuan Ke.

Shaughnessy, E. L. "Marriage, Divorce, and Revolution: Reading between the Lines for the *Book of Changes*." *The Journal of Asian Studies* 51.3 (1992): 594.

Shaughnessy, E. L. "The Origins of an *Yijing* Line Statement." *Early China* 20 (1995): 223–240.

Shen Jianhua 沈建華. "*Chu ju* Ruo ren yu Shangdai Ruo zu xintan" 《楚居》郮人與商代若族新探. In *Gudai jiandu baohu yu zhengli yanjiu*, ed. Qinghua daxue chutu wenxian yanjiu yu baohu zhongxin, Beijing daxue chutu wenxian yanjiusuo, Jingzhou wenwu baohu zhongxin, 213–218. Shanghai: Zhongxi, 2012.

Shen Jianhua. "Cong Qinghua jian *Chu ju* kan Dan Xi renwen quwei xingcheng" 從清華簡《楚居》看丹淅人文區位形成. In *Chu jian Chu wenhua yu xian Qin lishi wenhua guoji xueshu yantaohui lunwenji*, ed. Luo Yunhuan, 197–203. Wuhan: Hubei jiaoyu, 2013.

Shiji. See Sima Qian.

Shi Zhimian 施之勉, ed. *Hanshu jishi* 漢書集釋. Taipei: Sanmin, 2003.
Shouxian Cai Hou mu chutu yiwu 壽縣蔡侯墓出土遺物. Kaoguxue zhuankan 2.5. Beijing: Kexue, 1956.
Shuihudi Qin mu zhujian zhengli xiaozu 睡虎地秦墓竹簡整理小組, comp. *Shuihudi Qin mu zhujian* 睡虎地秦墓竹簡. Beijing: Wenwu, 2001.
Si Weizhi 斯維至. *Zhongguo gudai shehui lungao* 中國古代社會文化論稿. Yunchen congkan 允晨叢刊67. Taipei: Yunchen, 1997.
Sima Qian 司馬遷. *Shiji* 史記. Beijing: Zhonghua, 1959.
Song Jie 宋杰. "Handai Houfei 'jiu guan' yu 'waishe chanzi' fengsu" 漢代后妃 '就館' 與 '外舍產子' 風俗. *Lishi yanjiu* 6 (2009): 33–50.
Song Zhenhao 宋鎮豪, Duan Zhihong 段志洪, Chen Jianhua 陳建華, Cai Zhongmin 蔡忠民, and Tang Defeng 唐德風, eds. *Jiaguwenxian jicheng: jiaguexue tonglun* 甲骨文獻集成: 甲骨學通論. 40 vols. Chengdu: Sichuan daxue, 2001.
Su Jianzhou 蘇建洲. "Zailun Chu zhushu 'Zhouyi, Yi gua' 'rong' zi ji xiangguan de jige zi" 再論楚竹書《周易·頤卦》'融' 字及相關的幾個字. *Zhouyi yanjiu* 3 (2009): 36–39.
Su Xing 蘇興, ed. *Chunqiu fanlu yizheng* 春秋繁露義證. Beijing: Zhonghua, 1992.
Sui shu. See Wei Zheng.
Sukhu, G. *The Shaman and the Heresiarch: A New Interpretation of the Li Sao.* Albany: State University of New York Press, 2012.
Sun Min 孫敏. "Cong nüshen chongbai kan Chu wenhua nüxing siwei de xingcheng" 從女神崇拜看楚文化女性思維的形成. *Xinan minzu daxue xuebao* 8 (2006): 31–180.
Sun Yirang 孫詒讓 (1848–1908), ed. *Zhouli zhengyi* 周禮正義. 6 vols. Guoxue jiben series. Taibei: Taiwan Shangwu, 1967.
Sun Yirang, ed. *Mozi jiangu* 墨子閒詁. Zhuzi jicheng edition. Vol. 4. Shanghai: Shanghai shudian, 1986. Rpt. 1991.
Sun Zuoyun 孫作雲. "*Shijing* liange fawei" 《詩經》戀歌發微. *Shijing yu Zhoudai shehui yanjiu* 詩經與周代社會研究. Beijing: Zhonghua, 1966.
Taiping yulan 太平御覽. Beijing: Zhonghua, 1985. Rpt.
Takikawa Kametaro 瀧川龜太郎, *Shikikaichū kö shö* 史記會注考證. Taipei: Hongshi, 1977.
Takashima, Ken-ichi. *Studies of Fascicle Three of Inscriptions from the Yin Ruins.* 2 Vols. Special Publications no. 107B. Taipei: Institute of History and Philology, Academia Sinica, 2010.
Wang, J. *The Story of Stone: Intertextuality, Ancient Chinese Stone Lore, and the Stone Symbolism in Dream of the Red Chamber, Water Margin, and the Journey to the West.* Durham: Duke University Press, 1992.
Wang, R., ed. *Images of Women in Chinese Thought and Culture: Writings from the Pre-Qin Period through the Song Dynasty.* Indianapolis: Hackett, 2003.
Wang Fu (85?–163?). *Qianfu lun* 潛夫論. See Wang Jipei.
Wang Hui 王輝. *Shang Zhou jinwen* 商周金文. Zhongguo guwenzi daodu. Beijing: Wenwu, 2006.

Wang Jipei 汪繼培. *Qianfu lun jian jiaozheng* 潛夫論箋校正. Beijing: Zhonghua, 1985.
Wang Liqi 王利器. *Fengsu tongyi jiaozhu* 風俗通義校注. Beijing: Zhonghua, 1981.
Wang Qiang 王強. "Cong 'hushirenyou'kan wushu yanzhen de shehui yiyi" 從 "虎食人卣" 看巫術厭鎮的社會意义. Changsha: Changsha wenhua yichanwang, http://www.csswwj.gov.cn/bhcg/whycbhyj/201002/t20100223_219022.htm, 3/20/2014. Accessed at http://www.wenkuxiazai.com/doc/1ba27008bb68a98271fefa65.html on 2/26/2017.
Wang Rencong 王人聰. "Cai Hou X kao" 蔡侯X考. *Guwenzi yanjiu* 12 (1985): 321–326.
Wang Wei 王偉. "Qinghua jian *Chu ju* zhaji—Chu ren nüxing zuxian he gushi chuanshuo 清華簡《楚居》箚記——楚人女性祖先和古史傳說, www.gwz.fudan.edu.cn/, 6/9/2011.
Wang Xianqian 王先謙 (1842–1917), ed. *Houhanshu jijie* 後漢書集解. Beijing: Zhonghua, 2006.
Wang Xianqian (1842–1917), ed. *Hanshu buzhu* 漢書補註. Shanghai: Shanghai guji, 2009.
Wang Yinzhi 王引之. *Jingzhuan shici* 經傳釋詞. Nanjing: Jiangsu guji, 2000.
Wang Yunzhi 王蘊智. "'Yu,' 'hou' yuyuan ji bufen yahoo shechi yinshengmu tongbian guanxi hejie" '毓'、'后' 語源及部份牙喉舌齒音聲母通變關係合解. *Zhengzhou daxue xuebao* 1993.2. Rpt. in *Jiaguwenxian jicheng: jiaguexue tonglun* 甲骨文獻集成: 甲骨學通論, ed. Song Zhenhao 宋鎮豪, Duan Zhihong 段志洪, Chen Jianhua 陳建華, Cai Zhongmin 蔡忠民, and Tang Defeng 唐德風, vol. 14, 38–40. Chengdu: Sichuan daxue, 2001.
Wei Cide 魏慈德. "Qinghua jian *Chu ju* zhong Chu xianzu xiangguan wenti shilun—fulun Chu jian zhong 'X' fu" 清華簡《楚居》中楚先祖相關問題試論．—附論楚簡中的「X」符. *Chutu wenxian yanjiu shiye yu fangfa* 3出土文獻研究視野與方法 (第三輯). Taipei: Taiwan shufang 2012. 131–152.
Wei Zheng 魏徵, ed. *Suishu* 隋書. Beijing: Zhonghua, 1997.
Wen Yiduo 聞一多. "Gaotang shenü chuanshuo zhi fenxi" 高唐神女傳說之分析. *Shenhua yu shi* 神話與詩. Shanghai: Renmin, 2005. 69–96.
Wu, Yi-li. *Reproducing Women: Medicine, Metaphor, and Childbirth in Late Imperial China*. Berkeley: University of California Press, 2010.
Wu Yujiang 吳毓江, ed. *Mozi jiaozhu* 墨子校注. Beijing: Zhonghua, 2006.
Wu Yue Chunqiu 吳越春秋. Changsha: Yuelu Institute, 1996.
Wu Zhenfeng 吳鎮烽. *Shang Zhou qingtongqi mingwen ji tuxiang jicheng* 商周青銅器銘文暨圖像集成. Shanghai: Shanghai guji, 2012.
Xia Mailing 夏麥陵. "Qinghua jian *Chu ju* zhong Yitun he Fajian diwang shitan" 清華簡《楚居》中夷屯和發漸地望試探. In *Chu jian Chu wenhua yu xian Qin lishi wenhua guoji xueshu yantaohui lunwenji*, ed. Luo Yunhuan, 212–219. Wuhan: Hubei jiaoyu, 2013.
Xibei daxue wenbo xueyuan kaogu zhuanye, ed. 西北大學學院考古專業, *Fufeng anban yizhi fajue baogao* 扶風案板遺址發掘報告. Xibei daxue 211 gongcheng zhongdian zhichi xiangmu 西北大學211工程重點項目. Beijing: Kexue, 2000.

Xie, W. "Approaching the Dao: From Lao zi to Zhuang zi." *Journal of Chinese Philosophy* 27.4 (2000): 469–488.
Xie Weiyang 謝維揚. "Chu ju zhong Ji Lian niandai wenti xiaoyi" 《楚居》中季連年代問題小議. In *Chu jian Chu wenhua yu xian Qin lishi wenhua guoji xueshu yantaohui lunwenji*, ed. Luo Yunhuan, 151–155. Wuhan: Hubei jiaoyu, 2013.
Xu Lianggao 徐良高. *Zhongguo minzu wenhuayuan xintan* 中国民族文化源新探. Beijing: Shehui kexue wenxian, 1999.
Xu Shaohua 徐少華. "Gu Li guo lishi dili kaoyi" 古厲國歷史地理考異. *Lishidili* 歷史地理 19 (Shanghai renmin, 2003). In *Jing Chu lishi dili yu kaogu tanyan* 荊楚歷史地理與考古探研, 12–26. Beijing: Shangwu, 2010.
Xu Shaohua. "Ji Lian zaoqi judi ji xiangguan wenti kaoxi" 季連早期居地及相關問題考析. Qinghua daxue chutu wenxian yanjiu yu baohu zhongxin, ed. 清華大學出土文獻研究與保護中心編. *Qinghua jian yanjiu (di yi ji)—Qinghua daxue cang Zhanguo zhujian (yi) guoji xushu yantaohui lunwenji* 清華簡研究（第一輯）——《清華大學藏戰國竹簡（壹）》國際學術研討會論文集. Shanghai: Zhongxi, 2013. 277–287.
Xu Zhongshu 徐中舒. "Jinwen jiaci shili" 金文嘏辭釋例. In *Xu Zhongshu lishi lunwen xuanji* 徐中舒歷史論文選輯. Beijing: Zhonghua, 1998. 502–564.
Xunzi jijie 荀子集解. Shanghai: Shanghai guji, 1991.
Yao Xiaosui 姚孝遂 and Xiao Ding 肖丁, eds. *Yinxu jiagu keci leizuan* 殷墟甲骨刻辭類纂. 3 vols. Beijing: Zhonghua, 1989.
Yan Changgui 晏昌貴. *Wugui yu yinsi: Chujian suo jian fangshu zongjiao kao* 巫鬼與淫祀：楚簡所見方術宗教考. Chudi chutu Zhanguo jiance yanjiu Series. Wuchang: Wuhan University Press, 2010.
Yan Kejun 嚴可均 (1762–1843). *Quan shanggu sandai wen* 全上古三代文. Beijing: Shangwu, 1999.
Yan Ruxian 嚴汝嫻 and Song Zhaolin 宋兆麟. *Yongning Naxizu de muxizhi* 永寧納西族的母系制. Kunming: Yunnan renmin, 1983.
Yang Hua 楊華. "Xin Cai jidao jian zhong de liangge wenti" 新蔡祭禱簡中的兩個問題. *Jianbo* 2 (2007): 357–370.
Yates, R. "Medicine for Women in Early China: A Preliminary Survey." *Nan Nü* 7.2 (2005): 127–181.
Yin Difei 殷滌非. "Shouxian Cai Hou tongqi de zai yanjiu" 壽縣蔡侯銅器的再研究. *Kaogu yu wenwu* 4 (1984): 60–62.
Yin Hongbing 尹弘兵. "Chu ju zhong Chu xianzu de niandai wenti" 《楚居》中楚先祖的年代問題. In *Chu jian Chu wenhua yu xian Qin lishi wenhua guoji xueshu yantaohui lunwenji*, ed. Luo Yunhuan, 171–180. Wuhan: Hubei jiaoyu, 2013.
Yin Shengping 尹盛平. *Zhou wenhua kaogu yanjiu lunji* 周文化考古研究論集. Beijing: Wenwu, 2012.
Yinqueshan hanmu zhengli xiaozu 銀雀山漢墓整理小組. *Yinqueshan hanmu zhujian (er)* 銀雀山漢墓竹簡（貳）. Beijing: Wenwu, 2010.

Yu Xingwu 于省吾. "Shouxian Cai Hou mu tongqi mingwen kaoshi" 壽縣蔡侯墓銅器銘文考釋. *Guwenzi yanjiu* 1 (1979): 40–54.

Yu Xingwu. *Jiagu wenzi shilin* 甲骨文字釋林. Beijing: Zhonghua, 1996. Rpt. 1999.

Yuan Ke 袁珂. *Shanhaijing jiaoyi* 山海經校譯. Shanghai: Shanghai guji, 1985.

Yuan Ke. *Shanghaijing jiazhu* 山海經校註. Chengdu: Bashu, 1993.

Yuan Wenqing 院文清. "Chu boshu zhong de shenhua chuanshuo yu Chu xianzu puxi lüezheng" 楚帛書中的神話傳說與楚先祖譜系略證. Jingzhou bowuguan, ed. *Jingzhou bowuguan jianguan wushi zhounian jinian lunwenji* 荊州博物館建館五十週年紀念論文集. Beijing: Wenwu, 2008. 315–323.

Zhai Mailing 翟麦玲 and Zhang Rongfang 張榮芳. "Qing Han falü de xingbie tezheng" 秦漢法律的性別特徵. *Nandu xuetan* 4 (2005): 7–11.

Zhang Fuhai 張富海. "Shangbojian *Zigao* pian 'Hou Ji zhi mu' jiekaoshi" 上博簡《子羔》篇"后稷之母"節考釋. *Jianbo yanjiu wang*. www.jiabo.org, 1/17/2003.

Zhang Fuhai. "Chu xian 'Xue Xiong,' 'Yu Xiong' kaobian" 楚先'穴熊'、'鬻熊'考辨. *Jianbo* 5 (2010): 209–214.

Zhang Xiancheng 張顯成 and Zhou Qunli 周群麗. *Yinwan Hanmu jiandu jiaoli* 尹灣漢墓簡牘校理. Tianjin: Tianjin jiji, 2011.

Zhao Pingan 趙平安. "Cong Chu jian 'mian' de shidu tandao Jiaguwen de 'mian X'—fushi guwenzi zhong de 'ming'" 從楚簡"娩"的釋讀談到甲骨文的"娩X"——附釋古文字中的"冥." *Jianbo yanjiu 2001*. Vol. 1. Guilin: Guangxi shifan daxue, 2001. 55–59.

Zhao Pingan. *Xinchu jianbo yu guwenzi guwenxian yanjiu* 新出簡帛與古文字古文獻研究. Beijing: Shangwu, 2009.

Zhao Pingan. "*Chu ju* de xingzhi, zuozhe ji xiezuo niandai"《楚居》的性質、作者及寫作年代. *Qinghua daxue xuebao* 26.4 (2011): 29–33. Rpt. in *Gudai jiandu baohu yu zhengli yanjiu* 古代簡牘保護文獻與整理研究, ed. Qinghua daxue chutu wenxian yanjiu yu baohu zhongxin 清華大學出土文獻研究與保護中心, Beijing daxue chutu wenxian yanjiusuo 北京大學出土文獻研究所, Jingzhou wenwu baohu zhongxin 荊州文物保護中心, 178–184. Shanghai: Zhongxi, 2012.

Zhao Pingan. "Shishuo *Chu ju* 'yu chang yang'" 試說《楚居》xx羊. *Wenwu* 1 (2012): 75–76.

Zhao Pingan. "Shishi *Chu ju* zhong de yizu diming" 試釋《楚居》中的一組地名. Rpt. in *Gudai jiandu baohu yu zhengli yanjiu* 古代簡牘保護文獻與整理研究, ed. Qinghua daxue chutu wenxian yanjiu yu baohu zhongxin 清華大學出土文獻研究與保護中心, Beijing daxue chutu wenxian yanjiusuo 北京大學出土文獻研究所, Jingzhou wenwu baohu zhongxin 荊州文物保護中心, 172–177. Shanghai: Zhongxi, 2012.

Zhao Pingan. "Qinghua jian *Chu ju* Bi Wei, Bi X kao" 清華簡《楚居》妣隹、妣X考. In *Gudai jiandu baohu yu zhengli yanjiu*, ed. Qinghua daxue chutu wenxian yanjiu yu baohu zhongxin, Beijing daxue chutu wenxian yanjiusuo, Jingzhou wenwu baohu zhongxin, 185–190.

Zhao Pingan. "'San Chu xian' heyi bu baokuo Ji Lian" "三楚先" 何以不包括季連. *Handan xueyuan xuebao* 23 (2013): 62–65.

Zhao Rongjun 趙容俊. *Yinshang jiagu buci suojian zhi wushu* 殷商甲骨卜辭所見之巫術. Beijing: Zhonghua, 2011.

Zheng Xuan 鄭玄 (172–200). *Zhouli zhushu* 周禮注疏. In *Shisanjing zhushu*, vol. 1, ed. Ruan Yuan. Beijing: Zhonghua, 1980.

Zheng Xuan. *Yili zhushu* 儀禮注疏. In *Shisanjing zhushu*, vol. 1, ed. Ruan Yuan. Beijing: Zhonghua, 1980.

Zhongguo shehui kexueyuan kaogu yanjiusuo 中國社會科學院考古研究所. *Yinxu de faxian yu yanjiu* 殷墟的發現與研究. Kaoguxue zhuankan Series A23. Beijing: Kexue, 1994.

Zhongguo shehui kexueyuan kaogu yanjiusuo, comp. Yin *Zhou jinwen jicheng* 殷周金文集成. 18 vols. Beijing: Zhonghua, 1984–1994.

Zhongguo xueshu leibian 中國學術類編. *Shuowen jiezi gulin zhengbu hebian* 說文解字詁林補合編. 12 vols. Taipei: Dingwen, 1977.

Zhou Tianyou 周天游, ed. *Bajia Hou Hanshu jizhu* 八家後漢書輯注. Shanghai: Shanghai guji, 1986.

Zhou Yunzhong 周運中. "'Chu ju' Dong Zhou zhi qian dili kao"《楚居》東周之前地理考. In *Chu jian Chu wenhua yu xian Qin lishi wenhua guoji xueshu yantaohui lunwenji* 楚簡楚文化與先秦歷史文化國際學術研討會論文集, ed. Luo Yunhuan, 220–237. Wuhan: Hubei jiaoyu, 2013.

Zhu Junsheng 朱骏聲. *Shuowen tongxun dingsheng* 說文通訓定聲. Beijing: Zhonghua, 1984.

Zhu Xi 朱熹, ed. *Chuci jizhu* 楚辭集注. Shanghai and Hefei: Guji shudian and Anhui jiaoyu, 2001.

Zhu Zhenlei 祝振雷. "Anhui Shouxian Cai Hou mu chutu qingtongqi mingwen jishi" 安徽壽縣蔡侯墓出土青銅器銘文集釋. Jilin University, PhD dissertation, 2005–2006.

Zi Ju 子居. "Qinghua jian *Chu ju* jiexi" 清華簡《楚居》解析. Jianbo.org. http://www.jianbo.org/admin3/2011/ziju001.htm. Accessed 3/24/2015.

Index

Allan, Sarah, 16
almanacs, xii, 56, 57, 67, 121n28
  See also *Day Books*
ancestral spirits
  vs. abstractions, 45–46
  Chu, 3, 5–10, 63, 72, 75–92
  in *Chu ju*, 5, 6, 8, 71, 73–74, 90, 92
  Chu names for, xiii, 5–9, 10, 89–92
  female, 2, 3, 4, 22, 43, 53, 56, 69, 76–77, 79, 89–92, 93
  graphs for, 2–4, 38
  Shang, 1, 31, 32, 53, 76, 86–87, 97, 98, 100, 103, 107, 117n28
  Zhou, 23, 43–45
animals
  births of, 8
  in enclosures, 71–72
  in fertility symbolism, 13, 14, 15–16, 17
  gender of, 112n13
  sacrificial, 4, 9–10, 31, 33, 37, 47, 64, 72, 112n15
  See also bear; birds
Anyang (Henan), 1, 16, 76, 83, 102, 103
astral influences, 63, 66–68, 106
  and stem and branch system, 53, 56–59, 61–62, 67
astrolabes (*shipan*), 67

Ban *gui*, 112n5
Banpo culture (Shaanxi), 12
Baoxi, 90, 97
Bao *you*, 128n9
Baoshan divination texts, 73, 77, 121n23, 124n18
  on Chu ancestors, 5, 6, 8, 90
  graphs from, 5, 10, 125n21
Baoxi, 90, 91, 97, 128n12
Baozi *ding*, 26–27
"bear" (*xiong*), 5–7, 9, 92, 97, 112n7, 124n3, 126n29, 128n12
bell inscriptions, 6, 28–29, 77, 106, 124n5
Bi Gong (ritual site), 34–35, 41, 118n58
"Bi gong" (*Shijing*), 35
bigong (closed-off chamber), 71
Bin Gong *xu*, 118n52
birds, xiii, 8, 14–15, 17, 42, 60, 84
  Dark (*xuanniao*), 31–32, 33, 34, 41
birth
  cesarean, xii, 51, 73, 95, 130n42
  difficult, 69–70, 86, 92
  divine, 30, 40, 75–92, 94, 97, 98–101, 106, 109
  female experience of, xi–xiv, 11, 21, 54, 83, 103
  of females vs. males, xii, 2, 25, 33, 39, 53, 55–58, 59, 67, 120n26, 125n20

birth *(continued)*
  graphs for, 2–11, 16, 70, 111n5, 113n19
  place of, xii, 68–73, 101–2, 126n28
  pollution of, xii, 18, 69
  traumatic, xiii, xiv, 65, 70, 83–84, 86, 87, 93–107, 109
  and weaving, 46
birth, split-side (*xie sheng*), xii, 74, 125n26
  and Chu, 79–82, 84, 85, 87, 88, 92, 109
  geographic distribution of tales of, 93–94, 104, 106–7, 130nn42–43
  graphs for, 65, 79, 127n1
  of non-Zhou founders, 93–107, 109
  and shamans, xiii–xiv, 65–66
  and splitting imagery, 15, 16, 18, 103
  of twins, xiii, 65, 83, 96, 103–4, 128n1, 130n42
"Birth of the People" (Shengmin; *Shijing*), 30, 33, 38, 39–40, 94
body
  diagrams of, 60–63
  female, 9, 11–13, 18, 53–74
  graphs for, 1–3, 96
  split-open, 95, 99–100
  See also birth, split-side
bronze inscriptions, xi, 47
  on bells, 6, 28–29, 77, 106, 124n5
  in Cai Zhao Hou Shen tomb, 27–28, 47
  dowry, 26–27
  on female ancestors, 43, 77, 113n24
  on fertility, 16–17, 23–29
  graphs in, 3, 39, 114n7
  Shang, 16–17, 24, 95–96
  yin in, 95–96
  Zhou, 23–29, 43, 59, 76–77, 94, 95–96, 105
bronze vessels, 1, 4, 8–9, 15–16, 29, 76, 103
  See also particular vessels

Buddhism, 130n42

Cai, state of, 27, 28, 115n21, 116n22
Cai Yong, 32–33
Cai Zhao Hou Shen (Lord Shen of Cai) tomb, 27–28, 47, 115n21, 116n22
calendars
  in *Day Books*, 67, 120n5
  and divination, 21, 53–63, 125n20
Canhu people, 81, 86
"cave" (*xue*), xiii, 82, 84, 92, 102, 125n22
  in graphs, 5, 6, 7, 9, 10
celestial lodges (*su*), 67
Chang Pu, 79, 80, 89
Changyi (Fine Intention; Chu ancestor), 72, 75, 78–81, 88
  phonetics of, 89, 90, 91
Chanjing (*Ishinpō*), 49–51
Chen, state of, 77, 78
Chen Hou Yinzi *dui*, 75
Chen Huan, 35
Chen Mengjia, 30, 31, 117n28
Chen Shouqi, 35
Chen Wei, 71
Cheng, King (Zhou), 81, 86
Cheng Bo, 88
Cheng Tang, 32, 47, 106
child
  gender of, xii, 2, 24–29, 33, 39, 42, 53, 55–59, 67, 120n26, 125n20
  graphs for, 3, 9, 65, 69
Chinese University of Hong Kong bamboo slips, 129n16
Chong Li, 79, 81, 88, 89, 91
Chu, state of
  ancestral names in, 5–9, 8, 10, 89–92
  ancestral spirits of, 3, 5–10, 63, 72, 75–92
  birth tales from, 82–83, 87–88, 93, 97, 102–3, 105, 128n6

cultural geography of, 103, 105–6, 107, 122n41
deities of, 3, 7, 8, 9, 44, 76, 128n12
and fertility rites, 31–32
founders of, xiii, 3, 5–8, 10, 30, 65, 69–71, 76, 79–83, 85–88, 90, 92, 96–99, 102, 105, 111n5
gendered names in, 89–92, 105
graphs from, 5, 6–9, 122n44, 123n3
name ("thorn") of, xiii, xiv, 5, 70, 72, 73, 83, 84, 86, 88, 103, 104, 126n31, 127n38
and other states, 28, 78, 102, 103, 115n21
and Shang, 7, 8, 92, 93, 103, 104, 105–6
and split-side birth, 79–82, 84, 85, 87, 88, 92, 109
texts from, xi–xiv, 44, 61, 63
Chu Gongni bell, 6
Chu ju (Tsinghua University text), xi–xiv, 19, 42, 47, 61, 107
on Chu ancestors, 5, 6, 8, 71, 73–83, 86–89, 90, 92
on enclosures, 70–71, 72
graphs in, 6, 8, 10
on mothers, 43, 44, 45
on sequestering, 69–70
shamans in, 22, 83, 84, 87, 88, 126n31
on Shang, 105, 106
on split-side birth, xiii–xiv, 65, 94–96, 103, 104, 109
title of, 123n52
on Yu's birth, 100, 101, 102
"Chu shijia" (*Shiji*), 80, 86, 88
Chu Silk Manuscript, 19, 77, 96–97, 124n10
Chuci, 41, 93, 125n26
on Chu ancestors, 75, 83
on fertility rites, 31, 32
on Yu's birth, 98, 99, 102

Chunqiu, 103
Chunqiu fanlu, 93, 100
Chunqiu yuanming bao (Song Jun), 41
Confucianism, xi, 17, 36, 47, 94
"corpse" (*shi*), 2, 3, 122n44
curses, 2, 56, 61, 63–68, 69

Da Dai Liji, 75, 78, 79, 85, 88, 89
Da Meng Ji, 115n21
Dai, Lady, tomb of (Mawangdui), 100
Dao, 44, 45, 46, 47, 119n7
Dao, King (Chu), 73
Daodejing, 44–46, 119n5, 125n28
Daoism, 10, 22, 48
  "mother" in, 18, 44–45, 77, 117n41
"Dark Bird" (Xuanniao; *Shijing*), 31–34, 41
"darkness" (*ming*), 10, 113n17
Day Books (*Rishu*), xii, 73, 82, 83, 120n5
  body diagram in, 61–63
  Fangmatan, 8, 56, 57–58, 112n13
  Shuihudi, 42, 61–63, 67, 121n24, 126nn28–31, 127n38
day signs, 53, 58, 67
  See also stem and branch system
de (power, virtue, merit), 28, 44, 47, 73, 125n26
  and women, 34, 45
deities
  Chu, 3, 7, 8, 9, 44, 76, 128n12
  female, xii, 77
  and fertility rites, 22, 29–42
  See also ancestral spirits; Di; Huangdi; Shangdi; Taiyi; Tian
Dexter, Miriam, 15
Di (deities), 22, 63, 78, 114n7
  and fertility rites, 29–30, 40, 42
  and gender, 43, 44, 45
Di Ku, 32, 101–2
dipper, Northern, 67

divination, xii, 16, 74, 103
  on birth, 2, 22, 53–63, 67–68
  and calendars, 21, 53–63, 125n20
  and curses, 64–68
  stem and branch system in, 53, 56–59, 61–62, 67
  See also Baoshan divination texts; oracle bones
Diwang shiji (Huangfu Mi), 101
Dong *ding*, 77
Dongshanzui (Chaoyang City, Liaoning), 11
dowry inscriptions, 26–27
Dream of the Red Chamber, 100
"drinker" (*yin*), 5, 6, 92

embryonic transformation, 47–51
"enclosure," concept of, xii, 44, 47, 82, 94
  and birth graphs, 9–10
  and fertility images, 12, 16
  and sequestering, 70–72
Ersi Bi Qi *you*, 128n9
Erya, 40
exorcism, 2, 21, 38, 56, 64, 69
  and thorns, 73, 96, 104, 123n49, 126n31

Fengsu tongyi, 35, 79, 86, 89
fertility images, 11–19
  in Fu Hao tomb, 37, 76
  tigers in, 15–16, 17, 18
  and Yu's birth, 103
fertility rites, 25, 29–42, 128n3
  Gaomei, 22, 31–42, 71, 82, 98, 117n33, 118n48, 125n26
  and sexual symbolism, 13, 31, 37–39
  and shamans, 94
  Shang, 21–22
  sites of, 30–31, 32, 34, 37, 38, 40, 41, 71, 98
  and spring festivals, 36

  and thorns, 73
  Zhou, 23–29
Five Agents (*wuxing*), 32, 45, 48, 50, 56, 75, 101
Five Flavors, 48–49, 50
food
  influence of, 41, 67–68
  sacrifices of, 28, 29, 64
"form" (*zhuang*), 46–47
Fu Hao, 21–22, 54–55
  tomb of, 13–15, 16, 17, 37, 76
Fu Ju, 81, 88, 89, 91
Funing peoples, 39
Fuxi, 10, 19, 35, 77, 97, 100, 128n12
  and gender, 89–91

Gan Bao, 86–87, 88, 103, 105
Gaomei fertility rites, 22, 31–42, 82, 117n33, 118n48, 125n26
  sites of, 32, 34, 37, 38, 40, 41, 71, 98
Gao Xin (deity), 32, 35, 40
Gao Xin people, 101–2
Gao You, 36, 100
Gaoyang, 79, 80, 88, 91
  See also Zhuanxu
geomancy, 67, 70, 75
Gong Dian *pan*, 25
Granet, Marcel, 32, 36, 118n50
Guai Bo *gui*, 23–24
Guang, King (Wu), 27, 116n22
Guanzi, 36, 48–49
Gui people, 92, 107
Guifang people, 79, 130n43
Guizang, 99
Gun (father of Yu), 98–99, 102, 103, 124n3, 125n26, 126n29
Guo Moruo, 37
Guo Pu, 99
Guo Shu *fu*, 128n9
Guodian texts, 46, 106, 119n5

Han Liu, 126n30

Han period, xi, 107, 109, 111n1
  (Intro.)
 Chu genealogy in, 78–79, 82, 105
 deities in, 8, 32, 35, 44–45, 63,
  77–78, 94, 97, 100
 embryology in, 49–51
 fertility rites in, 31, 32–33, 36, 39,
  40
 fertility symbols from, 19, 39, 103
 Five Agents in, 45, 48
 graphs from, 9, 10, 35
 pregnancy in, 67, 68, 69, 96
 split-side birth tales in, 93, 98,
  100, 104
 trigrams in, 58, 61
 Yin and Yang in, 29, 68
 See also *Shiji*
Hanshu, 73, 79
Harper, Donald, 49
He Xin, 128n12
Hengxian (Eternal Prior), 45
hermaphroditic imagery, 13
homophones, 31, 46, 78, 104,
  116n24, 123n48, 128n1, 128n12
 and Di, 45, 119n3
Hongshan culture (Liaoning), 11–12
Hou Han shu, 101, 102
Hou Ji (deity), 30, 34–40, 94, 98,
  100, 103, 107, 128n3
Hou Mu Wu vessel, 16
Hu Houxuan, 22
Hu shi ren *you*, 114n28
Hu *zun*, 114n28
Huainanzi, 49–51, 93, 100, 121n27
Huaishen (*Ishinpō*), 49–51
Huaiyi peoples, 24
Huang Guohui, 112n5
Huangdi (Yellow Emperor), 32,
  123n1, 124n11, 125n23
 and Chu lineage, 75, 77–78,
  80–82, 88, 89, 91, 97
Huangfu Mi, 94, 101, 106
Hui people, 86, 88

India, 106–7, 130n42
Iroquois people, 104

Ji Lian (Chu progenitor), xiii, 10,
  70–72, 75, 79–92, 96, 102–5,
  122n38, 130n40
Jia Wen, 113n17
Jiaguwen heji, 21–22, 54–56
Jiandi (mother of Xie), 32, 87
Jiang Yuan (mother of Hou Ji), 30,
  34–40, 71, 94, 103
Jiao Mei (ritual site), 33, 34
Jin Jiang, 77
Jingzong (Chu Citadel Ancestral
  Shrine), 69–70, 71, 73, 83, 84,
  122n39
Journey to the West, 100
Ju, state of, 77

Kong Yingda, 33, 34
Kunwu people, 85

Lai bronzes, 76
Lao Tong ("Old Boy"; Chu ancestor),
  5–8, 79, 88–91, 125n21
Laozi (excavated texts), 44, 45, 46,
  119n5
Leizu, 79, 80, 89
Lewis, Mark E., 100
Li Ji, xiii, 84, 89, 90, 91, 104
Li Jiahao, 8
Li Xueqin, 122n44, 123n52
Liang period, 38, 39
Liangqi *ding*, 23
Lie, Ancestress (Liezu), xiii, 84, 88,
  91, 96, 103–4, 123n3
Liezi, 24–25
Liji (*Ritual Records*), 31, 33, 69,
  118n48
lineages, xii, xiii, 5, 11, 12
 Chu, 75–92
 Kong, 41
 Zhou, 23, 29–30, 76

Liu Hehui, 115n21
Liu Huan, 112n5
Liu Lexian, 121n20
Liu Xinfang, 95, 125n27
Liusheng *xu*, 24
Liuwan (Leduxian, Qinghai), 13
"Liyi zhi" (*Sui shu*; Wei Zheng), 38–39
loan words, 39, 113n16, 116nn23–25, 117n33, 119n3, 120n27, 125n26
  in birthing terms, 65, 111n5, 127n1
  in Chu ancestral names, 7, 9, 126nn29–31
  in place names, 30, 70, 118n48
Lu, state of, 34
Lu Cheng, 39
Lu Zhi, 33
Lu Zhong, 79–82, 85–89, 91, 92, 99, 107, 112n11, 128n12, 130n43
  See also Zhu Rong
Lunheng, 100, 103
Luo Xiaohua, 123n3
Lushi (Luo Mi), 35
Lüshi chunqiu, 36

Ma Chengyuan, 30, 117n33
Ma Guohan, 41
Ma Ruichen, 35
Mair, Victor, 15
Majiayao culture, 114n28
Manyi people, 92, 101–2
Mao Gong *ding*, 116n23
Mao Heng, 33, 34
Mawangdui texts, 49–51, 113n24
Mawangdui tomb, Lady Dai, 100
Mei Gong shrine, 35
Mi (Chu clan name), 81, 82, 84, 85, 86, 88, 89, 91
Miaodigou culture, 113n21
midwives, 9, 22, 83, 94
Mosou people, 41

mothers, xi, xii, 43–51
  ancestress, xiii, 15, 28, 29, 76, 77, 79, 82, 84, 88, 90, 91, 96, 97, 103–5, 109, 123n3, 125n26
  of Buddha, 107
  of Confucius, 40
  in Daoism, 18, 22, 44–45, 77, 117n41
  graphs for, 2, 3, 79, 85
  sequestering of, 68–72
  and silk, 46–47, 83
  split bodies of, xiii, 16, 18, 74, 79, 96, 99–100
  See also birth; Hou Ji; Ji Lian; pregnancy; Yu
Mozi, 37
music, 8, 28, 29, 47, 56, 112n13

Neolithic period, 1, 11–12, 13, 113nn20–21, 114n28
Nü Kui, 85, 86, 89, 91
Nü Tui, 85, 91
numerology, 56, 58–60, 62, 64–65, 129n19
Nüwa, 10, 19, 35, 77, 97, 100, 128n12
  and gender, 90–91

oracle bones (Shang), xii, 59, 107
  auspicious births in, 53–56
  on Chu, 5, 7, 105
  on curses, 63
  deities in, 44, 114n7
  on Fu Hao, 13, 15, 21–22, 54–55
  graphs from, 1–5, 7, 9–10, 39, 44, 71, 95–96, 123n3
  on sequestering, 69, 70
  yin in, 95–96
oral traditions, 7, 47, 79, 90, 102

Pan Geng, xiii, 84, 88, 92, 102, 105, 106

Pan Hu, 101–2
Pei Yin, 86–87
Peng Bangjiong, 22
Pengzu people, 86, 88, 89
phonetics
    of birth graphs, 10, 65, 102, 111n5, 127n1
    of Chu ancestral names, 7–8, 9, 89–92, 126nn29–31
    of Di and *de*, 45, 119n3
    and fertility rites, 30–31
    of "form," 46–47
    of Huang, 78
    See also homophones; loan words
Ping, King (Chu), 115n21
pollution, xii, 18
    and purification, 32, 56, 69, 118n50
pregnancy
    control of, 53–74
    divination on, 53–63
    graphs for, 2–3
    influences on, 63–68
    three-year, 86

qi (cosmic vapor), 37–38, 48, 56, 59–60, 68
Qi, state of, 26, 28–29, 73, 75, 77, 78, 106
Qi Hou *dui*, 26
Qianfu lun, 93, 101
Qin dynasty, 7, 111n1 (Intro.), 117n28, 126n31
    almanacs from, 56, 57, 67
    and Chu, 78, 88, 105, 106
Qing Shu *yi*, 26
Qiu Xigui, 97, 102

Rao Zongyi, 106, 121n20, 130n43
Raz, Gil, 49
Rongchengshi (Shanghai Museum text), 97, 126n29

Ruo people, 72

sacrifices
    of animals, 4, 9–10, 31, 33, 37, 47, 64, 72, 112n15
    annual (*yinsi*), 33–34, 38
    against curses, 64, 69
    and enclosures, 71–72, 107
    of food, 28, 29, 64
    graphs for, 71, 72, 122n44
    mei, 35–36
    to women, 2, 35
self-cultivation, 47–48, 100, 101
sequestering, 68–72, 73
sexual gatherings, 31–42
    See also Gaomei fertility rites
sexual symbolism, 11, 13–15, 18, 113n21
    and fertility rites, 13, 31, 37, 38–39, 41
    in graphs, 2, 4, 112n14
shamans, 121nn28–30, 123n3
    and birth, xiii–xiv, 9, 56, 65–66, 84, 87
    in *Chu ju*, 22, 83, 84, 87, 88, 126n31
    in *Day Book*, 67
    and fertility rites, 13, 17, 94
    as midwives, xiii, 9, 22, 83, 109
    and thorns, xiii–xiv, 73, 83, 84, 98, 126n31
Shan Zhouyao, 125n26
Shang dynasty, xii, 121n30, 129n37
    ancestors of, 1, 31, 32, 53, 76, 86–87, 97, 98, 100, 103, 107, 117n28
    birth tales of, 31, 32, 86–87, 94, 98, 100, 102, 103, 105
    bronze inscriptions from, 16–17, 24, 95–96
    and Chu, 7, 8, 81, 92, 93, 103, 104, 105–6

Shang dynasty (continued)
    deities of, 44
    and embryonic transformation, 47–48
    fertility rites in, 21–22, 24
    sequestration in, 69–71
    and splitting, 93, 95–96, 103
    Zhou term for (Yin), 83, 95–96, 105
    See also Fu Hao; oracle bones
Shangdi (High God), 78, 94, 116n28
    and fertility rites, 29, 30, 38, 40, 42
Shanghai Museum texts, 97, 106, 113n24, 121n21, 124n18, 126n29
    See also Zigao
Shangshu, 124n11
Shanhaijing (Classic of Mountains and Seas), 125n22, 126nn30–31
    on births, 93, 96, 98–99, 102
    on Chu ancestors, 7, 75, 79, 82, 83, 125n21
    and fertility rites, 31, 41–42
Shi Qiang pan, 76, 116n23, 128n9
Shiben, 97, 123n1, 123n52, 126n31
    on Chu ancestors, 75, 78, 79, 80, 85
Shifa (Tsinghua University text), 56, 58, 59–60, 121n13, 121n16, 128n1
    body diagram in, 60–61, 63
    on curses, 64–67
Shiji (Records of the Historian), 27, 30, 32, 115n21, 116n22
    on Chu ancestors, 75, 79–82, 85–89, 92
    on Huangdi, 123n1, 125n23
    Kong lineage in, 41
    on shrines, 70, 71
Shiji jijie (Pei Yin), 86–87
Shijing (Book of Odes), 40, 111n2
    (Ch. 1), 116n23, 116n26, 117nn41–43
    on bears, 112n7
    on births, 94–95

on enclosures, 71
on fertility rites, 31, 38
Mao commentary on, 33, 34
"Shengmin" in, 30, 33, 38, 39–40, 94
"Xuanniao" in, 31–34, 41
Shoushenji (Gan Bao), 87
Shu Yi bell inscriptions, 77, 106, 124n5
Shuogua (Explications of the Gua), 58–59, 65–66
Shuowen (Explicated Patterns; Xu Shen), 6, 9, 35, 50, 65
silk
    and motherhood, 46–47, 83
    texts on, xi, xii, 113n24
    See also Chu Silk Manuscript
Simu Wu ding, 114n28
social reproduction, 1, 15, 37, 53
    in Chu, 73, 79, 82
    and heirs, 43–44, 45
    women in, xii, 11, 74, 111n1 (Intro.)
    in Zhou, 25, 27, 29
Song, state of, 31, 106
Song Jun, 41
Spring and Autumn period, 7, 37, 73, 76–78, 105, 106
    fertility prayers in, 25–26, 28
stem and branch system (tiangan, dizhi), 53, 56–57, 59, 61–62, 67
Sui shu, 38–39
Sun Wukong (Monkey), 100

Taichan shu (Book of the Generation of the Fetus; Mawangdui), 49–51, 67, 121n17
Taiping yulan, 102
Taiyi (deity; Great Unity), 44–45, 47, 63, 77, 97
Taiyi Gives Birth to Water (Taiyi sheng shui), 44, 46, 63, 77
"Tang wen" (Liezi), 24–25

Tang zai Chimen (*Tang at Chi Gate*; Tsinghua University text), 47–51
thorns (*jing*), 123nn48–49, 129n37
  and birth, 73, 83, 84, 96, 98, 104, 126n31, 127n38
  and Chu, xiii, xiv, 5, 70, 72, 73, 83, 84, 86, 88, 103, 104, 126n31, 127n38
Tian (Heaven), 29, 32, 35, 44, 109, 116n28
transmitted texts
  on births, 30, 56, 98–99, 106
  on Chu ancestors, 77, 79, 82, 84, 90
  vs. excavated texts, xi, xii, 44–45, 99
  fertility prayers in, 23
  Fuxi and Nüwa in, 97
  on mothers, 44, 45–46
  See also particular titles
trigrams, 58–61, 64, 65, 66
Tsinghua University texts, xii, 47–51, 106, 123n52, 126n29
  See also Chu ju; Shifa
twins, xiv, 61, 67, 77, 94
  as Chu ancestors, 10, 42, 70, 82–83, 90, 92, 96, 127n39
  in non-Asian cultures, 92, 104, 130n42
  and split-side birth, xiii, 65, 83, 96, 103–4, 128n1, 130n42

Wang Chong, 103
Wang Jiang, 77
"Wang ju" (Shanghai Museum texts), 124n18
Wang Yi, 117n41
Wang Yinzhi, 117n33, 118n48
Wang Yunzhi, 113n24
Warring States period, 60, 105, 106
  Chu lineage in, 75, 78, 79
  and embryonic development, 47, 48

fertility rites in, 25, 29–42
graphs from, 3, 5, 6, 8, 10–11, 39, 46, 112n5
and split-side birth, 93, 97, 98, 102, 103, 107
Zhou lineage in, 29–30
  See also Zigao
Wei, Ancestress, xiii, 84, 88, 103, 125n26
Wei Yingqi (king of Qi), 78
Wei Zheng, 38
Wen, King (Zhou), 8, 28, 81, 82, 86
mother of, 29, 36
Wen Yiduo, 30, 31, 37
Wenzi, 49–51
Western Qiang people, 107, 130n43
Western Zhou period
  Chu ancestors in, 71, 76, 105, 122n41
  de in, 34
  deities in, 45, 94
  divination in, 58, 59
  female ancestors in, 76–77
  fertility rites in, 23–24
  graphs from, 2–3, 6, 7, 78, 95, 96, 113n25, 116n23
Wu, King (Chu), 90, 116n22
Wu, King (Zhou), 82
Wu, state of, 27, 28, 115n21
Wu Ding (Shang), 13, 21, 54, 69, 76
Wu Hui, 85, 88, 89, 91
Wu Yue chunqiu, 93, 100, 101
"Wudi benji" (*Shiji*), 80, 89
Wujing yiyi, 35

Xi Wangmu (Grandmother of the West), 48, 77, 119n18
Xia dynasty, 32, 47, 86, 93, 102, 107
Xian, Shaman (Wu Xian), xiii–xiv, 83, 84, 98, 126n31
Xie (sage-king; Shang ancestor), 97, 107
  birth of, 31, 32, 86–87, 98, 100, 103

Xin Cai texts (Henan), 5, 6, 7, 8, 77, 124n10
"Xingde xingshi" (Yinwan divination text), 127n36
Xinian (Tsinghua University text), 123n52
Xiong Li, 81, 88
Xiong Yi, 81–82, 88, 89
Xu Shen, 9
Xue Xiong (Chu ancestor), 5, 6, 79, 81, 88–92, 97, 127n42
Xue Yin (Chu ancestor), xiii, 5–7, 70, 82–84, 88–92, 95, 97, 103–5
Xunzi, 46, 83

Yangshao culture, 113n21
Yi peoples, 39
Yi Yin, 47
Yijing (*Zhouyi*; *Book of Changes*), 58, 61
  Shanghai Museum text of, 113n24, 121n21, 129n19
Yin. *See* Shang dynasty
Yin and Yang, 38, 63, 64, 67, 72, 75
  and divination, 56–57, 59–60
  in Han period, 29, 68
  and mother, 45, 47
Yin Shengping, 113n24
Yu (sage-king), 8, 86, 87, 97, 107, 111n5, 130n43
  birth of, 98, 102, 103, 125n26
Yu Xingwu, 96
Yu Xiong, 8, 10, 70, 71, 79, 81, 86, 88, 89
Yu Yin ("Birth Drinker"; Chu ancestor), 5, 6, 112n11
Yuan Wenqing, 128n12
Yuan Zhong, 88

"Yueling" (Monthly Ordinances; *Liji*), 31, 33, 118n48

Zeng Hou Yi tomb, 18, 19
Zhao Pingan, 113n17, 123n52, 126n28, 127n39
Zhejiang *zhong*, 116n23
Zheng Xuan, 31–32, 34–35, 38
Zhou dynasty
  ancestral spirits of, 23, 43–45
  birth tales from, 105
  bronze inscriptions from, 23–29, 43, 59, 76–77, 94, 95–96, 105
  and Chu, 70, 92, 93, 104, 122n41
  fertility prayers in, 23–29
  heirs in, 43–44
  lineage of, 23, 29–30, 76, 94
  and Shang, 83, 92, 95–96, 105
  social reproduction in, 25, 27, 29
Zhouli, 36
Zhouyi (Shanghai Museum text), 113n24, 121n21, 129n19
Zhu Rong ("Invoker Melder"; Lu Zhong; Chu ancestor), 5–8, 32, 75, 79, 81, 88, 112n11
  and Chu gendered names, 89, 90, 91, 92
Zhuangzi, 45
Zhuanxu, 79–82, 86, 88, 89, 91, 125n22, 126n30
Zigao (bamboo text; Shanghai Museum), 107, 117n35
  on births, 30, 40, 41, 96, 97–98, 100
  on fertility rites, 36, 37, 38
Zijing (Child Citadel; Shang), 69, 71
Zuojue wenzu *fangzun*, 24
Zuozhuan, 37, 68, 73, 83, 87, 115n21, 126nn28–29

www.ingramcontent.com/pod-product-compliance
Ingram Content Group UK Ltd.
Pitfield, Milton Keynes, MK11 3LW, UK
UKHW041919140426
5217IPUK00013B/234